Norris and Campbell's
Anaesthetics, Resuscitati

CW00548458

For Churchill Livingstone:

Publisher: Timothy Horne
Project Editor: Janice Urquhart
Copy Editor: Kathleen Orr
Indexer: Nina Boyd
Project Controller: Kay Hunston
Design Direction: Erik Bigland

Norris and Campbell's
Anaesthetics, Resuscitation and Intensive Care

Sir Donald Campbell CBE MBChB FRCA FRCP (Glas and Edin) FRCS (Edin and Eng) FFARCSI
Professor Emeritus, University of Glasgow;
Honorary Consultant Anaesthetist, Glasgow Royal Infirmary,
Glasgow, UK

Alastair A. Spence CBE MD FRCA FRCP (Glas and Edin) FRCS (Edin and Eng) Hon FDS, RCS Eng
Professor of Anaesthetics, University of Edinburgh;
Honorary Consultant Anaesthetist, Royal Infirmary of
Edinburgh, Edinburgh, UK

EIGHTH EDITION

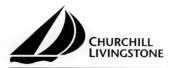

CHURCHILL
LIVINGSTONE

NEW YORK EDINBURGH LONDON MADRID MELBOURNE
SAN FRANCISCO TOKYO 1997

CHURCHILL LIVINGSTONE
Medical Division of Pearson Professional Limited

Distributed in the United States of America by Churchill
Livingstone Inc., 650 Avenue of the Americas, New York,
N.Y. 10011, and by associated companies, branches and
representatives throughout the world.

First edition 1965
Second edition 1968
Third edition 1971
Fourth edition 1974
Fifth edition 1978
Sixth edition 1985
Seventh edition 1990
Eighth edition 1997

ISBN 0 443 04886 X

British Library Cataloguing in Publication Data
A catalogue record for this book is available from the British
Library

Library of Congress Cataloging in Publication Data
A catalog record for this book is available from the Library of
Congress

Medical knowledge is constantly changing. As new
information becomes available, changes in treatment,
procedures, equipment and the use of drugs become
necessary. The authors and the publishers have, as far as it is
possible, taken care to ensure that the information given in the
text is accurate and up to date. However, readers are strongly
advised to confirm that the information, especially legislation
with regard to drug usage, complies with current and
standards of practice.

The
publisher's
policy is to use
**paper manufactured
from sustainable forests**

Produced by Longman Singapore Publishers (Pte) Ltd
Printed in Singapore

Contents

Preface to the Eighth Edition

This edition takes the book to its fourth decade of publication. As always the pace of change has necessitated radical revision in places and the introduction of new chapters. Pharmaceutical development has had a major impact on intravenous induction, with propofol (Diprivan) becoming more widely used than thiopentone in some settings. There is yet another generation of neuromuscular blocking drugs — rocuronium and mivacurium — and two new inhalation anaesthetics in desflurane and sevoflurane.

In the last edition we described recovery care in the knowledge that a minority of centres did not have recovery rooms and that ad hoc arrangements in operating theatres and surgical wards were sitll occurring. Happily that is in the past, and now change focuses on the high dependency unit with the concept of 'progressive patient care' better understood if not fully realized. Day-case anaesthesia blossoms as does the organized approach to better postoperative pain relief with many hospitals offering an Acute Pain Service.

Throughout clinical medicine the search is on for evidence based practice with guidelines which bring a consistent, more structured and safer practice than was possible previously. That influence applies to some forms of intensive care, to anaesthesia, in day-case surgery, monitoring, pain relief and resuscitation. Audit is also part of the vocabulary and we have seen benefit from local initiatives and also national schemes such as the Confidential Enquiry into Perioperative Death and the Confidential Enquiry into Maternal Mortality. Critical incident reporting is becoming an established part of anaesthetic and intensive care work.

1996 marks the sesquicentenary of the first successful public demonstration of ether anaesthesia by W. T. G. Morton who gave ether in Boston in October 1846. The first anaesthetic in Europe was given on 19th December 1846 in the dental practice of James

Robinson, at Gower Street, London. From the beginning of anaesthesia two figures dominated the scene. John Snow, a Yorkshire doctor, trained in Newcastle-on-Tyne and practised in London. He studied and wrote brilliantly on ether, developing a science from an art. Sir James Young Simpson was Professor of Midwifery at Edinburgh. He took an early interest in ether with the special intention of attempting to relieve the pain of labour; from the beginning of ether anaesthesia Simpson was in close communication with Snow. Simpson's major contribution, however, was the introduction of chloroform anaesthesia in 1847. These two great figures contributed more than anaesthetic practice. Snow discovered that cholera was a water borne disease (ahead of the identification of microbes). Thus he is a founding figure in public health medicine. Simpson founded the specialty of gynaecology and, like Snow, campaigned about the risks of 'hospitalism' — the occurrence of fatal sepsis as a feature of overcrowded and badly designed hospitals. Simpson was vilified for attempting to relieve labour pain with anaesthesia because fundamentalists within the Church held that to be against God's will. In 1857, however, Queen Victoria received chloroform from John Snow at the birth of Prince Leopold and immediately analgesia in labour was held to be respectable. Snow made a major contribution to developing the use of chloroform anaesthesia. He and Simpson made continuing contributions to the science of anaesthesia for the rest of their lives.

In the centre of Boston there is a memorial to Morton and to ether, erected in 1867, and which incorporates the inscription: 'BEFORE WHOM in all time Surgery was Agony'. Modern anaesthesia and perioperative care seem almost infinitely sophisticated compared with the beginnings in 1846. The basic ethos remains the same.

Donald Campbell

1996   Alastair A. Spence

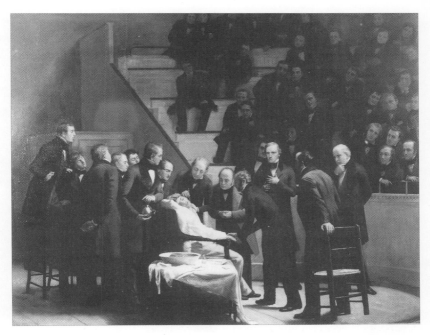

'The First Operation under Ether' — painted in oils between 1881 and 1894 by Robert C. Hinckley and owned by the Boston Medical Library.

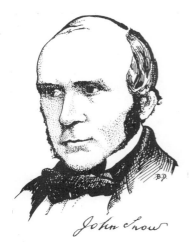

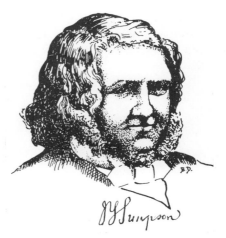

John Snow 1813–1858.   James Young Simpson 1811–1870.

Preface to the First Edition

The administration of anaesthetics in this country is now firmly established in the hands of the specialist anaesthetist. Indeed after qualification a doctor may never require to give an anaesthetic again if he does not wish to do so. Most doctors, however, in their hospital life and indeed outwith hospital, will at some time work in co-operation with members of the anaesthetic department staff. Surgeons, obstetricians and dentists, of course, are in daily contact with anaesthetists, physicians are meeting and working with them in the treatment of various chest diseases, and many other specialists also co-operate with them.

To the student we hope to offer a background to his practical teaching in the operating theatre and explain the 'whys' of anaesthesia rather than to attempt to explain how to give an anaesthetic. If he wishes to learn how to give an anaesthetic, he must do this in the operating theatre and over the course of many weeks or even months. We hope also to show that the interests and work of the anaesthetist are not limited to the operating theatre.

To the resident in hospital we hope to explain how he may help the anaesthetist and thus his patients by careful preoperative care of the patient and by thinking of the therapy he is using and the effect it may have on the anaesthetic later. We hope also he will realise that there are many ways in which the anaesthetist can help him and that there are times when he should call a consultant anaesthetist rather than a consultant surgeon or physician.

In many hospitals the resident will find himself dealing with patients in intensive care units, particularly those dealing with respiratory emergencies, both medical and surgical. This is a field of work where it is essential that everyone should know what is expected of him and what can be done to help severely disabled patients. It is essential that 'the man on the spot' should be fully conversant with all the methods which are used.

No matter what path the student intends to follow, we feel that a thorough knowledge of methods of resuscitation will prove invaluable to him whether he practises in hospital, in general practice or in any other branch of medicine. Acute respiratory and cardiac failure may occur anywhere and the chance of survival of the patient depends entirely on the ability of those present to maintain or restart an efficient circulation and ventilation within a few minutes.

It is for this reason that we have dealt with resuscitation, intensive care, tracheal intubation and intravenous therapy in greater practical detail. As with the administration of anaesthetics, however, there is no substitute for practical training and experience.

Finally, we feel that a knowledge of the accidents and medico-legal hazards which are associated with anaesthesia, resuscitation and intensive care will impress on both students and residents the need for care in applying these techniques.

Glasgow, 1965   W. Norris
                                                     D. Campbell

Acknowledgements

We wish to thank Mrs Cynthia Middleton for her substantial secretarial help with this revision.

We are grateful to the following colleagues for their assistance: Drs G. M. R. Bowler, B. Cook, A. M. D. Crean, I. T. H. Foo, Anne S. Goldie, D. Justins, Nicola J. Maran, M. J. Souter, C. M. Thorpe, J. G. Thomas, J. J. Wedgwood and Miss Marilyn Young.

We wish to thank Association of Anaesthetists, British Journal of Anaesthesia, European Resuscitation Council, Abbott Laboratories, Portex for permission to copy material in their possession or copyright.

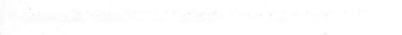

1. Basic concepts

Analgesia means absence of pain and is a term used to describe the state in which pain has been abolished but other sensations remain and the patient is conscious. *Anaesthesia* means absence of all sensation, touch, temperature, posture and pain. The patient may be unconscious, having apparently lost all sensation, or the term may apply to nerve block affecting a region of the body.

The conduction of painful impulses to the brain from a site of injury may be interrupted at one of several points between the origin and the sensory cortex. We are concerned with the use of drugs which do this, although in injury, or some surgical procedures for the permanent relief of pain, nerves may be cut or tracts in the spinal cord divided. Such permanent intervention might be used to treat the pain of incurable malignant disease. Tumours themselves may interrupt the passage of impulses by producing ischaemia. Extreme cold can block nerve conduction also.

Some drugs may relieve pain without having their dominant effect on the nervous system. For example, salicylates ease pain by reducing inflammation, and cytotoxic drugs by causing regression of tumour.

GENERAL ANAESTHESIA

Modern techniques of anaesthesia are often complex in respect of both the range of drugs and the equipment used. However, it is best to begin by considering the simple and traditional method of producing anaesthesia with a single drug. A large number of drugs are capable of abolishing all sensation but some, such as methyl alcohol, can be expected to produce permanent tissue damage while others, such as ethyl alcohol, although less damaging to tissue, are associated with prolonged and unpleasant recovery. The relatively small group of drugs known as the *inhalation anaesthetics*,

1

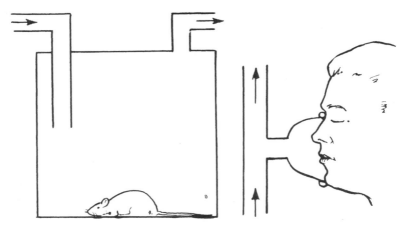

Fig. 1.1   Diagram to show simple anaesthetic techniques for mouse and man.

for example halothane or enflurane, produce reversible depression of the central nervous system with a quality of recovery that is acceptable to the patient.

Figure 1.1 shows examples of simple inhalation techniques for a mouse and a man respectively. In both cases the primary objective is to achieve a sufficient concentration of anaesthetic in the central nervous system so that the mouse or man will not move in response to a stimulus such as incision of the skin. In both examples the inspired gas (the gaseous environment) must contain not only molecules of the anaesthetic but a concentration of oxygen sufficient to maintain life. Moreover, the expired carbon dioxide must not contribute significantly to the next breath. Thus the inspired gas must be as 'fresh' as possible for each breath.

The transfer of anaesthetic molecules to the brain occurs via the lungs and the pulmonary and arterial circulation. Of course, the anaesthetic is distributed to all the tissues of the body in addition to the central nervous system. Although this is inevitable, in many instances it is undesirable as many anaesthetics have known adverse side-effects such as myocardial depression. The transfer of molecules from one phase to another (gaseous environment to lung, lung to blood, etc.) can occur only if there is a *partial pressure* or *tension* gradient from one phase to another (Fig. 1.2). In a gas mixture the partial pressure of one of the components is the product of its percentage concentration and the total ambient pressure. Thus at normal atmospheric pressure (101.3 kPa or 760 mmHg)

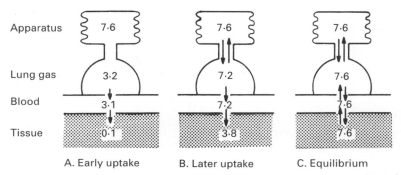

Apparatus	7·6	7·6	7·6
Lung gas	3·2	7·2	7·6
Blood	3·1	7·2	7·6
Tissue	0·1	3·8	7·6
	A. Early uptake	B. Later uptake	C. Equilibrium

Fig. 1.2 A. An early phase of inhalation anaesthesia in which the lung and blood partial pressure of the anaesthetic (halothane in this case) is less than that of the delivery system (apparatus) but greater than that of the blood or tissue. Net transfer is in one direction. B. The lung and blood have almost equilibrated with the delivery system but tissue lags behind. Net transfer continues. This represents the condition during most anaesthetics. C. Equilibrium has occurred across all compartments and there is no net transfer. This condition is never achieved in practice since periods of anaesthesia of even many hours would be too short.

the partial pressure of 1% of halothane will be 1 kPa approximately. The partial pressure or tension of gases in liquid such as blood or other tissues may be defined as the partial pressure which that gas would exert in a gas mixture which is in equilibrium with the liquid. When the transfer of gas molecules across the various phases of the body is complete there is partial pressure equilibrium. Thereafter, although molecules continue to move at random from one phase to another there is no *net* exchange from one phase to another.

Uptake and elimination patterns

Figure 1.3 shows the pattern of uptake to equilibrium by the lung alveoli and brain following the administration of five inhalation anaesthetics. Note the different rates at which the partial pressure in brain approaches equilibrium with a partial pressure in the inspired gas. Although there are many reasons for the differences between these uptake curves, the dominant factor is the difference in blood solubility, nitrous oxide being poorly soluble and diethyl ether being highly soluble. A similar set of curves can be produced for the elimination of these agents when the inspired partial pressure has been restored to zero (the anaesthetic has been discontinued), the poorly soluble agents being eliminated rapidly.

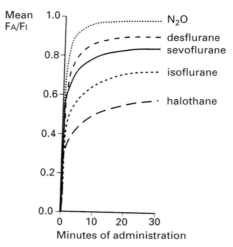

Fig. 1.3   Time course of changes in the lung alveolar concentration of five inhalation anaesthetics related to the inspired concentration which is $F_1=1.0$.

Figure 1.4 shows a family of theoretical curves for the uptake of halothane to equilibrium at three different inspired partial pressures. The interrupted line shows the uptake pattern which might occur during the administration of an anaesthetic and illustrates the inspired partial pressure set initially to a higher level than that with which the brain needs to equilibrate, so that brain concentration reaches the required level faster than is possible if the inspired concentration were maintained at a constant value throughout. Giving a large 'loading' dose is familiar in many types of drug administration, for example digitalization. The accepted term for this in anaesthetic practice is *overpressure*.

Potency and dosage; the concept of MAC

Doctors are accustomed to thinking of the administration of drugs in terms of a recommended dose range and it may be asked how the dose of an inhalation anaesthetic can be determined. Consider a situation in which the tissues of the healthy patient are in equilibrium with a known partial pressure or tension of halothane which causes just sufficient depression of the brain that the patient does not move in response to incision of the skin. The concentration of halothane in the brain tissue, determined by the tension and the solubility in the brain of halothane, may be calculated and exoff 2 3 4 5 6 7 8 9 10 11

off 2 3 4 5 6 7 8 9 10 11 12

off 2 3 4 5 6 7 8 9 10 11 12 13

off 2 3 4 5 6 7 8 9 10 11 12 13 14

off 2 3 4 5 6 7 8 9 10 11 12 13 14 15

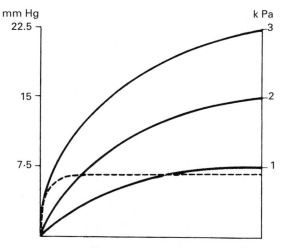

Fig. 1.4 Family of curves showing progress towards equilibrium of a body tissue (brain for example) for three different inspired tensions of halothane (vertical axis mmHg or kPa). The interrupted line shows what is likely to occur during administration of a typical anaesthetic when the vaporizer is set first to a high value and reduced gradually.

pressed as mmol/100 g brain. It is perhaps reassuring to know that the anaesthetist does not undertake such calculations routinely! However, the important point is that approximately the same mean (± a narrow scatter) concentration of halothane in the brain of any patient in a similar state of health will produce the same depth of anaesthesia. Indeed, as a general rule the same concentration would probably produce about the same depth of anaesthesia in many other species, for example in the mouse which we considered earlier.

It can be shown for halothane that the inspired concentration which we have been considering is 0.75–0.8% at sea level or 6 mmHg (0.8 kPa) at any altitude. This is called the minimum alveolar concentration for halothane (MAC). At high altitude, where the total pressure is lower, the percentage must be increased to allow the same partial pressure as we considered at sea level. If the total ambient pressure were greater than at sea level, the concentration needed would be less. It is *partial pressure* (or tension) that matters.

All the inhalation anaesthetic agents have MAC values, the significance of which is the same as in the example of halothane. Some of these values are given in Table 1.1. There is an approxi-

Table 1.1   Some properties of the inhalation anaesthetics

Anaesthetic	Boiling point °C	MAC % of 1 atm.	Partition coefficients	
			Blood : gas	Oil : gas
Sevoflurane	58.5	2.0	0.6	53
Enflurane	56.5	1.7	1.9	96
Halothane	50.0	0.8	2.3	224
Isoflurane	48.5	1.2	1.4	91
Diethyl ether	35.0	1.9	15.0	91
Desflurane	23.0	6 to 9	0.42	18
Nitrous oxide	−89.0	105.0	0.47	

mately inverse linear relationship between MAC for an inhalation anaesthetic and its lipid solubility (Fig. 1.5). Traditionally 'lipid' solubility relates to olive oil taken as representing (but not of course the same as) the lipids of brain.

Those who are mathematically minded will have realized that the depth of anaesthesia would appear to depend on the molecular concentration of the anaesthetic in the brain, rather than on any individual property of one drug as compared with another. Thus MAC is the best description of the dose value of an inhalation

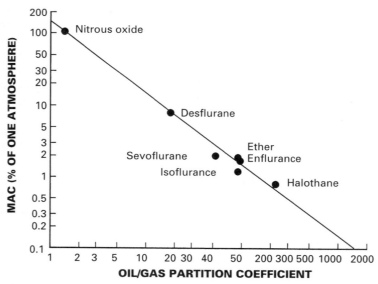

Fig. 1.5   Relationship between oil : gas partition coefficient (an index of lipid solubility) and MAC for seven anaesthetic agents.

anaesthetic. It must be remembered, however, that MAC presumes equilibrium between brain and inspired gas. We have already outlined the events preceding the state of equilibrium. Among other factors, we have seen that the time necessary to achieve concentration, or tension, close to the equilibrium value varies greatly between agents, being relatively short for nitrous oxide, long for diethyl ether, and for halothane somewhere between these two. Such considerations may be very important in determining the suitability of a drug in a specific clinical situation.

We are now in a position to consider what is meant by the *potency* of an inhalation anaesthetic. Textbooks of pharmacology are often rather confusing about this matter, implying that some molecules have a more potent effect on the brain than others. We have explained why this is unlikely to be so.

A drug such as nitrous oxide (MAC = 106.6 kPa) which has a low lipid solubility must be given in high concentrations to achieve any obvious clinical effect. Indeed, surgical anaesthesia cannot be produced with nitrous oxide even at the maximum partial pressure obtainable at normal atmospheric pressure. Thus there are limitations to the use of nitrous oxide as an anaesthetic and it may be described loosely as having a low potency when compared with halothane (MAC = 0.8 kPa). However the discerning reader will realize that this is a reflection of solubility in tissues rather than an intrinsic pharmacological action of the molecules.

Fractions of MAC may be combined. Thus, as an approximation, one-half of the MAC value of nitrous oxide—53 kPa (approximately 50% at sea level)—combined with one-half of the MAC value of halothane—0.4 kPa (0.4%)—will provide surgical anaesthesia when equilibrium between inspired gas and brain has been achieved.

The components of anaesthesia

Anaesthesia has three components: unconsciousness, analgesia and muscular relaxation. In the past it was common practice to produce all three by the administration of potent inhalation agents such as diethyl ether and it is also possible to do this with other volatile anaesthetics. Since the unconscious patient does not 'feel' pain in the normally accepted sense, but shows reflex responses to it, 'analgesia' is often replaced by 'suppression of reflex activity' in the triad. It is in this context that the term 'analgesia' is used in this book when we are considering the unconscious patient. By using small doses of specific drugs to produce separately hypnosis, analgesia and muscle relaxation, it is possible to provide the appropriate combination for each patient.

Hypnosis

It is usual to induce unconsciousness by intravenous injection of a drug which has a short duration of action. Thiopentone and propofol are the most popular agents but there are others. Alternatively unconsciousness can be induced within an inhaled mixture of nitrous oxide with oxygen to which has been added an anaesthetic vapour. During anaesthesia hypnosis is maintained by inhalation of anaesthetic gases. Some anaesthetists attempt maintenance with intravenous infusion of propofol which has a relatively short pharmacological half-life. Thiopentone has a long half-life and is not suitable for this purpose although it was tried in the past.

Analgesia

Inhalation anaesthesia produces a degree of analgesia and nitrous oxide is particularly effective, although any volatile agent given to accompany nitrous oxide will confer a degree of analgesia. In many methods of anaesthesia the anaesthetist is likely to give short- or long-acting opioids. Where a patient is expected to breathe spontaneously throughout the surgical procedure particular care is needed in the choice and dosage of opioid so as to avoid undesirable ventilatory depression. In patients undergoing artificial ventilation the contribution of the opioid to an anaesthetic may be greater, through a higher dose, because immediate considerations of respiratory depression are unimportant. It is important, however, in these circumstances to ensure that, when a patient is restored to spontaneous breathing at the end of the operation, no unwanted residual effects of the opioid persist.

Muscle relaxation

Some degree of muscle relaxation is necessary for most operations. It eases surgical access and minimizes the amount of tissue trauma caused by stretching. This may vary from simple relaxation of the forearm muscles during manipulation of a Colles' fracture to the more profound muscular paralysis needed for upper abdominal and intrathoracic operations. Although muscle relaxation can be produced by the use of one of the more potent volatile anaesthetic agents, the quantities which would be needed to achieve profound relaxation may cause delayed recovery or risk toxicity. Therefore, one of a range of myoneural blocking drugs (sometimes called neuromuscular blockers) may be given. These act by antagonizing the effect of acetylcholine at the muscle endplate. A consequence of their use is failure of the muscles of breathing. Thus, artificial ventilation has to be instituted by intermittent positive pressure (see p. 166), usually applied via a tracheal tube.

The introduction of tubocurarine (curare), the first neuromuscular blocker to be used clinically, brought the need for a wide range of skills in respiratory care and detailed understanding of pulmonary and cardiovascular physiology. The growth of anaesthesia as a specialty, and the later involvement of the anaesthetist in respiratory intensive care, stemmed primarily from this development.

Although the terms 'myoneural blocker' or 'neuromuscular blocking drug' are correct for this class of drug they are usually loosely referred to as 'muscle relaxants' in everyday practice. Without wishing to be tediously semantic, we feel it is worth noting that a variety of drug actions can produce muscle relaxation, including inhalation anaesthetics as noted above, but only the neuromuscular blockers have such a specific effect on the neuromuscular junction.

Mode of action of anaesthetics

No one knows precisely how the drugs which produce general anaesthesia act or whether they all act at the same site or sites within the central nervous system, although there are many theories. Elucidation of this complex problem remains one of the great challenges to medical science and is the subject of active research programmes by many pharmacologists and anaesthetists throughout the world.

LOCAL OR REGIONAL ANAESTHESIA OR ANALGESIA

Local anaesthetic drugs

The passage of impulses along nerves is associated with electrical changes. Sodium and potassium ions enter and leave the nerve during the different phases of conduction and this ionic migration takes place at the nodes of Ranvier, constrictions in the myelinated nerves at intervals of about 1 mm. The action potential resulting from the migration of these ions extends from one node to another and thus the impulse passes along the nerve. Although the mechanism is not fully understood, local anaesthetic drugs stabilize the nodal membrane to prevent permeability to ions, and this interferes with the passage of impulses along the n :rve.

Local anaesthetic solutions are stored fc ˙ injection as water-soluble salts, usually the hydrochloride. Such solutions are acid, having a low pH. When injected, they come in contact with tissues which are alkaline (pH about 7.4) and this is sufficient to cause a reaction which liberates the base of the local anaesthetic (which is required for stabilization of the membrane). If a solution is injected into an infected area where the pH is low—5.6 or less—the salt will fail to liberate base. This accounts for the failure of local anaesthetics to act in the presence of infection.

Topical application (Fig. 1.6)

Local anaesthetic solutions may be painted or sprayed on mucous membranes or wound surfaces. They are absorbed locally and produce analgesia in the area to which they have been applied. This method is not effective when the solution is applied to unbroken skin as the drug is not absorbed and does not reach the nerve endings.

Topical analgesia may be used for examinations or minor surgical procedures of the urethra, nose, throat and bronchial tree. In the preparation of a wound for cleansing and local infiltration it may be helpful to begin by using a swab which has been soaked in a dilute solution of a local anaesthetic.

EMLA is the commercial name given to a 'eutectic mixture of

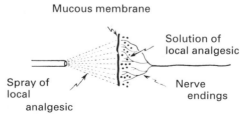

Fig. 1.6   Topical application.

local anaesthetics' (lignocaine and prilocaine). When this is applied to the skin from a special adhesive pad there is slow absorption through skin with onset of anaesthesia over a period of about 1 hour. In a eutectic mixture the two local anaesthetic molecules act together, almost as a new compound, although there is no modification of the molecular structures.

EMLA is particularly useful in young children before intravenous cannulation.

Local infiltrations (Fig. 1.7)

Injection of a dilute local anaesthetic solution in the area of the proposed operation will block the perception of pain at the level of the nerve endings. This is perhaps the simplest method of analgesia and is used widely for minor surgical operations. If restricted to this type of case it is a safe procedure and has few, if any, after-effects so that the patient is able to eat and drink and return home shortly after the operation. The method can be used for more extensive operations but larger doses of the drug are necessary and side-effects are more likely. Extensive infiltration is an unpleasant procedure for the patient. It is a common fallacy that local infiltration using dilute anaesthetic solutions is an entirely safe procedure. This is true only when two safeguards are observed. First, great care must be taken to avoid administering an overdose. It is easy to forget that in extensive procedures considerable quantities of the drug may have been injected, although in dilute solution. Care must be taken to avoid intravascular injection of these drugs. Before and at intervals during the infiltration of the area of operation, aspiration with the syringe must be performed regularly to ensure that the needle does not lie within a blood vessel. (Local anaesthetic agents have toxic properties as have other drugs and an overdose could be lethal.)

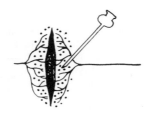

Fig. 1.7   Local infiltration.

Infiltration is an excellent method for the surgeon working without the assistance of an anaesthetist. Provided that the safeguards described are observed carefully, the technique is almost without complications. The method should not be used in the presence of local infection and care should be taken to prevent the anatomy of the area becoming distorted by the injection; this may happen, for example, if an excessive volume of solution is injected in proximity to a vein before cannulation.

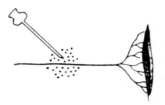

Fig. 1.8   Regional nerve block.

Nerve block (Fig. 1.8)

The main nerve which supplies the area of an operation can be blocked by injecting a local anaesthetic solution close to it. Thus it is possible, with a few injections, to produce analgesia for a wide area. This is achieved by using quite small doses of the drug and may be less harmful than widespread infiltration. The technique has the advantage that the solution may be injected some distance proximal to the site of operation so that distortion of structures is avoided and the presence of sepsis at the operative site is not a contraindication. The technique is of particular value when the nerves which supply an area are easily accessible. With this method, as with those which follow, the presence of a bone structure as a landmark in positioning the tip of the needle improves the chance of success. For example, the first rib is a convenient landmark in supraclavicular block of the brachial plexus (p. 220). For attempts to block the sciatic nerve, there are no bone structures immediately adjacent to the nerve and failure is more frequent.

Paravertebral nerve block (Fig. 1.9)

In this method the nerves are blocked close to the vertebrae, before the sympathetic fibres have left the main nerve. This technique is

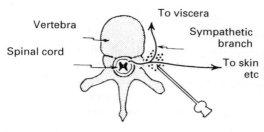

Fig. 1.9   Paraventral nerve block.

used rarely for surgical procedures inside the abdomen. It may be useful for blocking nerves such as those innervating a leg, to produce sympathetic block and vasodilation in vascular disease.

We will consider two techniques which, by one single injection, may produce analgesia over a wide area of the body.

Spinal or subarachnoid analgesia (Fig. 1.10)

A local anaesthetic solution introduced to the cerebrospinal fluid may distribute widely to affect a large number of nerves. In this way, by a single injection, analgesia, muscular relaxation and sympathetic blockade affecting a large part of the body may be produced easily.

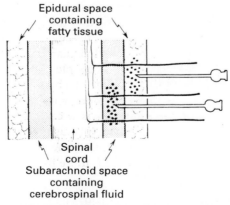

Fig. 1.10   Epidural and spinal analgesia: the diagram illustrates the two sites at which the analgesic solution may be deposited, following introduction of the needle through the intervertebral space.

The technique has many advantages:

- Excellent analgesia
- Complete muscular relaxation
- Sympathetic blockade which produces not only a reduction in arterial pressure, advantageous in reducing heamorrhage at the operative site, but also a contracted bowel which allows easy access to all parts of the abdomen
- Easy estimation of volume of solution which will produce a given area of analgesia
- It is possible, though undesirable, for one person to perform the subarachnoid block and then perform the operation. The practice, however, may be fully justified in underdeveloped societies where medical skills are very scarce.

A disadvantage of spinal anaesthesia is that most patients prefer to be asleep during the operation, particularly in countries in which the services of trained anaesthetic personnel are easily available. For this reason spinal nerve block may be performed for its special advantages, along with a light general anaesthetic.

In the past, spinal anaesthesia has been associated with a number of complications. Transient nerve palsy and headache are still relatively common. Other complications, though rare, can be very severe, including paraplegia which has followed spinal analgesia, even when given by competent anaesthetists, using apparently impeccable techniques. Headache may last for several days. This may be a result of a leakage of cerebrospinal fluid through the lumbar puncture, and can be minimized by using a fine needle (25 gauge). Paraplegia has been attributed to many causes: infection, trauma, chemical irritation or the use of unsuitable solutions.

Whilst it is right to draw attention to the complications and difficulties of spinal anaesthesia, there are many circumstances in which the method is invaluable (see Ch. 15).

Extradural or epidural analgesia (Fig. 1.11)

Most of the advantages of spinal analgesia without some of the complications may be obtained by extradural or epidural analgesia (the terms are synonymous).

As they leave the subarachnoid space the nerves pass through the adjacent extradural space, which is filled with fatty tissue and connects with the paravertebral spaces. By injecting a local anaesthetic solution into the extradural space it is possible to obtain con-

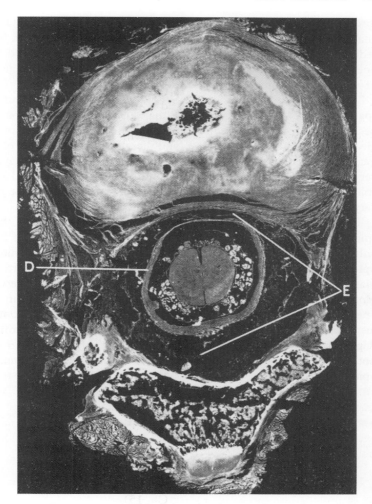

Fig. 1.11   Transverse section of spine between first and second lumbar vertebrae. E is the epidural space and D the dura and arachnoid mater separating it from the subarachnoid space.

ditions identical to subarachnoid blockade, namely good analgesia, sympathetic blockade and good muscle relaxation. The risk of introducing infection to the subarachnoid space and the possibility of direct damage to the spinal cord is eliminated and, because the arachnoid membrane is not punctured, headache is unlikely. It is possible to pass a catheter into the extradural space and inject through it, at intervals, repeated doses of the analgesia solution. This enables analgesia to be continued into the postoperative period; by reducing postoperative pain, deep breathing is facilitated and post-operative chest complications may be avoided. This method is also of value in producing pain relief during labour (see p. 199).

The main disadvantages of the technique are that the extradural space is more difficult to identify than the subarachnoid space because the former is a potential space like the pleural cavity. For a given extent of block, the volume (and therefore the total dose) of a local anaesthetic which must be injected to the extradural space is very much greater than would be required for subarachnoid or spinal anaesthesia. It should be noted that paraplegia, although very rare, has followed the use of this technique.

The discovery of opiate receptors in the dorsal horn area of the spinal cord has led to many attempts to produce pain relief by either subarachnoid or extradural injection of solutions containing opioids. Highly lipophilic opioids, such as diamorphine, are partic-ularly effective. Analgesia results without the risk of motor nerve block, and these techniques have been used to relieve pain after operation and the intractable pain caused by cancer. In some instances, however, the patient may suffer unexpected respiratory depression of unpredictable and late onset. Itching of the skin is not life-threatening but may be a tedious complication of spinal opioids.

2. Drugs used in anaesthesia

INHALATION ANAESTHETICS

Most of these are volatile liquids at room temperature and require to be vaporized in a carrier gas. The exception is nitrous oxide which exists as a gas at room temperature and pressure but is stored mainly as a liquid at high pressure in a cylinder.

Important distinguishing characteristics

- *Solubility in blood and lipid phases of the body.* High blood solubility will result in prolonged uptake to equilibrium and a prolonged recovery.
- *MAC value.* A high MAC value (see also p. 4) may limit the depth of unconsciousness which can be achieved with the drug, having regard to the need for oxygen at an alveolar pressure not less than 29 kPa (220 mmHg) and the presence of carbon dioxide 5.3 kPa (40 mmHg) and water vapour 6.2 kPa (47 mmHg).
- *Muscle relaxation.* This refers to the extent to which anaesthesia with the agent is accompanied by muscle relaxation, thus aiding surgical access.
- *Volatility.* A substance with a high boiling point will be difficult to vaporize.
- *Irritation of the respiratory tract* will limit the ease with which anaesthesia can be induced.
- *Effect on vital functions.* In depressing the brain most agents depress the respiratory centre also. Excessive respiratory depression causes hypoventilation of the lung alveoli with consequent retention of carbon dioxide in the tissues and the risk of hypoxaemia.
- *Serious cardiac arrhythmia* is more likely with some agents than

with others. This risk may be enhanced in the presence of increased concentrations of adrenaline, either endogenous, for example as a result of hypoxia or hypercarbia, or injected in the course of the surgical procedure.

- *Other undesired effects* such as involuntary movements during surgery, nausea, vomiting or shivering in the postoperative period.
- *Toxicity.* Some agents may be associated with damage to organs such as the liver or kidney. Such effects may be either a direct effect of the drug itself or may result from the formation of metabolites of the drug molecule.
- *Flammability and risk of explosion* when mixed with oxygen. Most agents presenting this problem have been removed from practice. The exception is diethyl ether which remains of value in some of the developing countries. There is a need to avoid surgical diathermy and to work only with full antistatic features in anaesthetic and operating areas.
- *Compatibility with chemicals used for absorbing carbon dioxide in a circle system.* Some substances may decompose to form poisonous products.
- *Compatibility with other drugs* such as adrenaline.
- *Availability.* Some drugs may be unavailable because of high cost. Nitrous oxide in cylinders must be transported from factory to hospital and there may be difficulty in obtaining supplies in remote areas.

Nitrous oxide has been known for more than 200 years. It is sometimes called 'laughing gas' because one of its early uses was as a music hall entertainment (Fig. 2.1). It is pleasant to inhale and non-irritant. It has no obvious adverse effect on the vital organs although exposure to nitrous oxide lasting for more than 24 hours causes significant oxidation of vitamin B_{12}. This has theoretical implications for disturbance of folate metabolism although the practical implications in clinical anaesthesia are negligible. There are reports of serious incapacity from neuropathy, similar to sub-acute combined degeneration of the spinal cord, in individuals who have persistently abused nitrous oxide.

Nitrous oxide is poorly soluble in the tissues and its MAC value is just in excess of one atmosphere (105 kPa). Thus anaesthesia without hypoxaemia is not possible with nitrous oxide alone unless in a hyperbaric environment. In spite of these limitations nitrous oxide is the most commonly used inhalation anaesthetic. Its poor

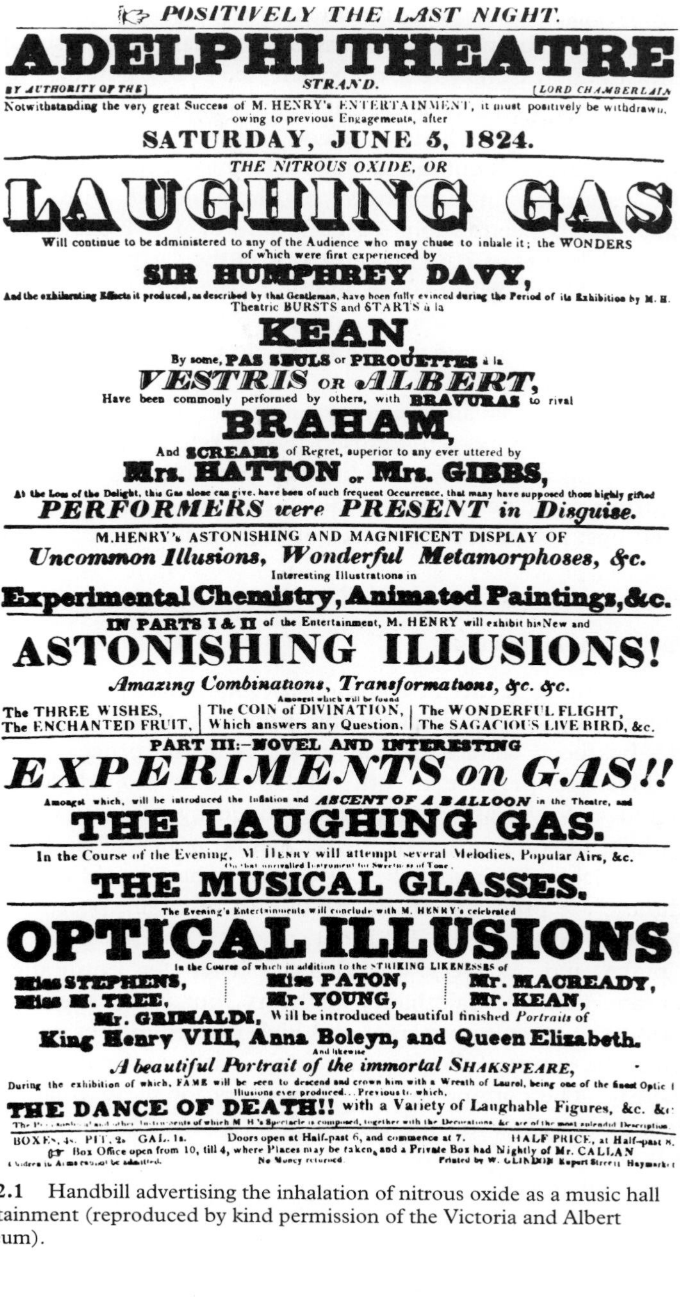

Fig. 2.1   Handbill advertising the inhalation of nitrous oxide as a music hall entertainment (reproduced by kind permission of the Victoria and Albert Museum).

solubility ensures a rapid onset of, and speedy recovery from, its effects and the absence of side-effects is of great value. It should be given with not less than 30% of oxygen (see p. 23) and this mixture is often used as a carrier gas for a suitable volatile agent.

Consider a patient who is to receive enflurane anaesthesia for the repair of a hernia. If enflurane is the sole anaesthetic it would need to be vaporized in a mixture of air enriched with oxygen. Equilibrium concentrations of enflurane of 1.7–2.0% might be required. The use of 70% nitrous oxide in the carrier gas (approximately 0.7 MAC) with oxygen and no nitrogen reduces the necessary enflurane concentration to about 0.6%. Since the side-effects of enflurane may be undesirable (see below) this reduced concentration is preferable.

Nitrous oxide is an excellent analgesic. Concentrations not exceeding 50% in oxygen are used for the relief of pain in labour, in the postoperative period and in the intensive care unit. In first aid nitrous oxide has proved invaluable in accident and other first aid settings; a significant number of paramedics are trained in its use.

Volatile anaesthetics

There are three agents in common use: halothane, enflurane and isoflurane. Desflurane is attracting growing interest. Sevoflurane, which has been widely used in Japan, is in the process of being introduced to practice in other relatively developed countries. Preferences for volatile agents are dictated by a variety of factors including, in some hospitals, departmental policy. Halothane has been available for more than 40 years whereas enflurane and isoflurane are products of the 1970s. All three are potent anaesthetics (see under MAC, Table 1.1).

Uptake and recovery are slightly faster for enflurane and isoflurane than for halothane, in theory, but isoflurane is rather irritant to the respiratory tract and high concentrations cannot be given at the outset of the procedure if the patient is breathing spontaneously. The commonly used vaporizers for these volatiles deliver a maximum concentration of 5% (5 volumes per cent) and this is particularly limiting in the case of enflurane which is less potent (higher MAC) than the other two agents.

All three drugs are powerful respiratory depressants and reduce the arterial pressure. In the case of halothane the hypotension is a combined result of reduced cardiac output and peripheral resistance, whereas reduced peripheral resistance is the dominant factor in the case of isoflurane. Enflurane depresses the myocardium less than does halothane.

Halothane may slow the heart rate; nodal rhythm, and sometimes atrial and ventricular extrasystole are a sign of overdose. It also sensitizes the heart to the arrhythmogenic effect of circulating catecholamines, whether endogenous or injected. Enflurane and isoflurane are much less likely to cause arrhythmia and are to be preferred if adrenaline is to be injected for any reason.

An important factor in the choice of volatile is the stability of the molecules and the possible implications for toxicity. About 20% of the tissue content of halothane will be metabolized, the remainder being excreted unchanged through the lungs at the end of the procedure. While the normal products of metabolism (biotransformation) are known to be non-toxic, there is a possibility of abnormal patterns with the production of metabolites that may induce liver injury. Halothane hepatitis is an accepted entity, although very rare. The aetiology of the condition is not well understood but it is thought that it is more likely to occur if halothane is given twice to a patient within a period of 3 months. Although the matter is scientifically controversial, many anaesthetists have abandoned the use of halothane in practice because of concern about this rare complication.

About 40% of the body content of enflurane is biotransformed and free fluoride is produced which may, in theory, produce renal damage. Enflurane is contraindicated in patients with renal failure although it has never been properly established that enflurane has demonstrable nephrotoxicity. In contrast, isoflurane is a very stable compound, less than 0.1% of the tissue content being metabolized, and its principal benefit to many anaesthetists is its freedom from the stigma of organ toxicity.

Occasionally enflurane causes involuntary muscular movements associated with an epileptiform EEG pattern. There are no after-effects from these neurological side-effects, but the drug is considered unsuitable for patients suffering from epilepsy.

All three volatiles produce a significant degree of muscle relaxation at deeper levels of anaesthesia which is usually desirable. During recovery, however, there may be muscle rigidity and there may be a shivering or shaking pattern in the period leading up to the patient becoming fully responsive. This phenomenon is associated with a heavily increased demand for oxygen, and oxygen enrichment of the inspired gas should be given.

Desflurane

Desflurane is a halogenated ether introduced to anaesthetic practice in 1990. It is a very stable compound with low solubility in blood and fat. Its cardiorespiratory effects are similar to those of isoflurane. Its boiling point is comparatively low and a new design of vaporizer has been necessary for its use. Of all the inhalation anaesthetics the drug is thought to have the least risk of organ damage. Its main benefit is a fast onset and offset of effect which is regarded by some as important when fast recovery from anaesthesia is necessary. The vapour causes some irritation to the respiratory tract. At the time of writing the place of desflurane in anaesthetic practice is not yet established, mainly because of high cost, the special vaporizer, and the fact that the speed of effect is not so dramatically different from the older drugs as to have a clear clinical benefit.

Sevoflurane

This compound has been known for 25 years. Like desflurane it has low solubility. Its cardiorespiratory effects are similar to those of isoflurane. The drug has been used successfully in Japan for a number of years and is making something of a comeback in western countries where previous interest was confined to research studies. Sevoflurane is expensive and, like desflurane, is most likely to be used in a circle or rebreathing system with soda lime to absorb CO_2 and to reduce cost (see p. 47). There is unresolved controversy as to whether sevoflurane becomes dangerously unstable in contact with soda lime if the temperature of the soda lime becomes very high. At the time of writing this is seen as a theoretical rather than a practical disadvantage.

Diethyl ether (ether)

This was the most widely used of the volatile anaesthetics for many years. In industrialized countries it has been abandoned, except for very occasional use in children. It is inexpensive and easily available and these factors, coupled with the recognized safety of ether, make it an attractive drug in the less developed countries. MAC is 1.9%, the vapour is extremely irritant to breathe and bronchial and salivary secretions may be alarmingly copious, especially if atropine has not been given as a premedicant. Breath holding, coughing and laryngeal spasm during induction of ether anaesthesia call for skill in its administration. The drug is highly soluble in blood so that induction tends to be prolonged. On the other hand, the risk of accidental overdose is remote. Ether stimulates the sympathetic nervous system and the cardiac output is well maintained. At deep levels of anaesthesia with ether muscle relaxation is excellent. Respiratory depression is rare. Nausea and vomiting are common after ether and may be protracted. Ether is inflammable in mixtures with air and *explosive* when the concentration of oxygen exceeds that in air.

Ether was introduced in 1846 by W.T.G. Morton in Boston. That event is generally recognized as the discovery of anaesthesia for painless surgery. Because chloroform was more potent than ether it was hailed by many throughout the world as an advantage over the Boston development and some considered that it was chloroform, rather than ether, which led to the widespread popularity of inhalation anaesthesia. The down side, of course, was an increased risk of accidental overdose and death from chloroform because of its greater potency.

Chloroform

Since the last edition of this book a number of volatile anaesthetics have disappeared from use and need not be discussed. For historical and sentimental reasons we leave a few comments on chloroform because the 150th anniversary of its introduction by Sir James Young Simpson falls in 1997. Chloroform was a powerful anaesthetic and relatively non-irritant with a profile which was in many respects similar to that of halothane. In the early part of the twentieth century, however, it became unpopular because of the risk of fatal cardiac arrhythmia and fear of hepatoxicity in the postoperative period. If chloroform had been introduced to modern anaesthetic practice as a new compound it might have had a better reputation but the availability of several better modern drugs makes its use in current practice inappropriate. It is associated with a high incidence of postoperative nausea and vomiting.

Oxygen

Oxygen must be given in all anaesthetic techniques. If air is used as the carrier gas the concentration will be 21% approximately but greater concentrations are normally desirable in an anaesthetic mixture.

During anaesthesia, either with the patient breathing spontaneously or where ventilation is controlled, oxygen transfer from the
lungs to the blood is impaired. A number of factors may cause this
(Fig. 2.2), notably an alteration in the ventilation/perfusion ratio in
the lung (increased physiological 'shunt'), where perfusion is relatively greater in the dependent parts of the lung at the expense of
upper parts, or ventilation is relatively greater in the upper parts at
the expense of the dependent parts. In ventilation/perfusion disturbances both of these processes may occur together.

Depression of the cardiac output may lead to excessive desaturation of the blood returning to the lungs. The shunted fraction of
this being mixed with normal oxygenated blood from the pulmonary capillaries has the effect of reducing the 'mixed' PO_2.
During controlled ventilation, unless large tidal volumes are used,
some areas of the lung may be underventilated, leading to arterio-
venous 'shunting' of blood.

While these mechanisms are complex, it should be stressed that
the percentage of oxygen administered during anaesthesia should
seldom be less than 30% as this has been shown to compensate for
the factors mentioned and to produce an arterial oxygen tension of
at least 13.3 kPa (100 mmHg) in healthy subjects.

When suitable apparatus or supplies of nitrous oxide and oxygen
are not readily available, the use of air as a carrier gas for a volatile
agent may be necessary; for example ether may be given with air in
unsophisticated circumstances. Adding additional oxygen to the

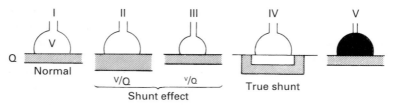

Fig. 2.2 Diagrammatic representation of shunt effect and true shunt within the
lung. Example I shows the normal relation of ventilation to perfusion which will
give optimum oxygenation of the blood in an air-breathing subject. Examples II
and III represent regions of the lung in which perfusion is excessive in relation to
ventilation. This will cause suboptimal oxygenation of blood unless the alveolar
Po_2 is increased by increasing the inspired oxygen concentration. In examples
IV and V true shunt has occurred and the alveolar gas has no influence on the
perfusing blood. Thus oxygen therapy will be of little use except that, by effecting
an increase in the oxygen content of blood leaving the more normal alveolar units
in other parts of the lung, the effect of a true shunt may be counteracted to a small
extent.

carrier air is likely to overcome any difficulties of arterial oxygenation but in the case of ether renders the inhaled mixture explosive. Depending on the working circumstances it may be more sensible for the patient to be rendered mildly hypoxaemic for a brief period than for the environment to be such that the whole operating team and the patient are at risk of being blown up!

Volatile anaesthetics can be administered in carrier gas mixtures carrying very high concentrations of oxygen (90% or more). This may be justified in some emergency settings but for many patients there may be adverse effects from breathing high concentrations of oxygen: nitrogen is washed out from the alveoli and replaced by oxygen which is absorbed rapidly and patchy collapse of lung alveoli may occur. It should also be remembered that patients with chronic lung disease who exist normally on a 'hypoxic drive' may suffer acute ventilatory depression when the inspired oxygen tension is excessive.

If there are closed air-containing cavities in the body (e.g. middle ear surgery), the anaesthetist may wish to avoid using nitrous oxide as the carrier gas because the diffusion of nitrous oxide with the cavity risks expansion or a build up of pressure. Most modern anaesthetic machines are designed to meter air with oxygen.

Carbon dioxide

The therapeutic administration of carbon dioxide during anaesthesia was popular and useful over many years. Concentrations of 5% of carbon dioxide added to the inspired gas, to stimulate breathing, were of value during anaesthesia, particularly with diethyl ether or other irritant vapours. After artificial ventilation of the lungs some patients may be hypocapnic as a result of excess CO_2 being washed from the body tissues. Addition of CO_2 to the inspired gas was helpful in creating the conditions for the return of spontaneous breathing. In spite of these benefits, mishaps resulting from the inadvertent use of carbon dioxide, with serious risk to the patient, have led to the removal of CO_2 supplies from many anaesthetic machines.

INTRAVENOUS ANAESTHETIC AGENTS

These include the intravenous induction agents and also a number of drugs given by intravenous injection which may be used alone or in combination with inhalation anaesthetics to maintain anaesthesia during operation.

The usefulness of an intravenous anaesthetic is determined by the following important factors:

- *Speed of onset of action.* All of the drugs in regular use render the patient unconscious within seconds.
- *Speed of recovery.* This may be rapid, as in the case of some of the induction agents, or prolonged, as in the case of some of the long-acting narcotic analgesics used to maintain anaesthesia. A knowledge of the likely period for onset of action and recovery helps to indicate the appropriate drug in a given situation.
- *Disposal in the body.* If the drug is detoxicated or excreted rapidly, full recovery from its effect will occur early. Such a drug may be given repeatedly with little risk of accumulation.
- *Quality of anaesthesia.* Some drugs may produce sleep, although being poor analgesics, while others may cause profound analgesia with sleep occurring only at very high doses. Anaesthesia induced by an intravenous anaesthetic may be associated with undesirable side-effects such as coughing, hiccough or involuntary movements.
- *The likelihood of depression of the cardiovascular system and the respiratory system.* The 'therapeutic ratio' is the dose required to produce anaesthesia related to the amount which is associated with severe cardiovascular and respiratory depression, or other undesirable effect.
- *Ease of administration.* Some drugs may cause pain on injection and damage to veins, or tissue injury in the event of extravascular injection.
- *Convenience of preparation.* Some compounds are stable in solution, while others have to be dissolved in water immediately before administration.
- *Risk of hypersensitivity reactions.* This relates particularly to anaphylactoid responses.
- *Compatibility with other drugs likely to be administered during the anaesthetic.* In recent years there have been reported anaphylactoid reactions which could not be attributed to individual drug molecules themselves. This has led to a hypothesis that, on occasion, complex chemical interactions may occur, for example within the lumen of indwelling cannulae.

Thiopentone sodium

The sulphur analogue of pentobarbitone, this is supplied as a yellow powder with a bottle of sterile water sufficient to make a 2.5% solution. As the yellow powder contains 6% sodium carbonate to stop the formation of (insoluble) thiopentone acid, the solution has a high pH (10.4–10.6). The solution is prepared immediately before use as it is relatively unstable and is not normally kept for longer than 24–48 hours. Thiopentone, like other barbiturates, causes sedation and induces sleep but has no analgesic activity. Indeed it has been shown in some studies to have an anti-analgesic effect. This is responsible for some of the postoperative restlessness which is found in patients in whom anaesthesia has been induced with thiopentone and in whom unrelieved pain is a prominent postoperative feature. Thiopentone is generally regarded as unsatisfactory when used as the sole anaesthetic.

Thiopentone depresses the respiratory centre. After a deep breath or even a yawn respiration is reduced, mainly in amplitude. Apnoea may supervene for a few moments then breathing restarts, shallow but regular. Surgical and other stimuli such as venepuncture may increase the depth of breathing during this period.

A decrease in arterial pressure usually accompanies the injection of thiopentone though this can be minimized by slow injection. The effect is largely a result of vasodilation of the peripheral vascular bed and is transient, as a rule, provided that only small doses of the drug have been given. The autonomic nervous system is depressed, the sympathetic more than the parasympathetic. The relative parasympathetic overactivity may cause laryngeal spasm, bronchospasm, coughing and bucking during induction of anaesthesia.

Recovery from a single 'sleep dose' of thiopentone is rapid, mainly because of redistribution of the drug in the body, thus reducing the concentration in the central nervous system. After recovery of consciousness the redistributed drug is gradually returned to the blood and metabolized in the liver. Small quantities of barbiturate can be detected in the blood 24 hours after administration of thiopentone. It is for this reason that thiopentone is not particularly suited to outpatient anaesthesia because there is a protracted hangover effect. The breakdown products are excreted via the kidney and in patients with renal insufficiency the drug should be used with extreme caution.

The solution of thiopentone is extremely alkaline and, if it is injected into subcutaneous tissue or, worse, into an artery, severe damage may result. These complications are dealt with when considering intravenous induction of anaesthesia (p. 113).

Despite the introduction of newer intravenous anaesthetics,

notably propofol, thiopentone is still widely used in anaesthetic practice.

Methohexitone sodium

A methylated oxybarbiturate, this is used as a 1% aqueous solution (pH of 11.1). The time to both wakening and complete recovery is much shorter than after thiopentone and there is little hangover effect. In the past the drug was popular in outpatient anaesthesia, notably for dental procedures. Some patients who receive injections of methohexitone intravenously complain of pain at the site of injection or along the course of the vein during injection, despite the fact that the intravenous cannula is correctly positioned within the vein.

There is a high incidence of hiccough and of muscular movements and twitching following administration of methohexitone. Introduction of propofol anaesthesia has considerably reduced the need for methohexitone.

Propofol

Marketed under the trade name Diprivan, propofol is a di-isopropylphenol presented in a soyabean oil emulsion. The dose for induction of anaesthesia is approximately 2.5 mg/kg. The drug is a potent respiratory depressant and can cause marked reduction in arterial pressure. Propofol is rapidly cleared from the circulation and the speed of recovery from its effect is of great value in patients undergoing day-case surgery and in others who are required to be as alert as possible after the administration of anaesthesia has ended. On injection of propoful some patients complain of pain or discomfort. This can be reduced by adding dilute local anaesthetic solution with the injection, although many anaesthetists do not regard the problem as sufficiently serious to justify that.

The short half-life of propofol has attracted its use as a continuous infusion to maintain anaesthesia throughout the surgical procedure. It is usual to add other drugs, such as opioids or nitrous oxide, as part of this type of anaesthetic technique. The technique of establishing a state of surgical anaesthesia using intravenous drugs, often given by infusion, and avoiding inhalation anaesthesia altogether has enjoyed a certain fashion and is known as *total intravenous anaesthesia.*

Other intravenous anaesthetic agents

Ketamine (Ketalar), a powerful analgesic, may be given to induce anaesthesia. It produces a state of dissociation short of unconsciousness with preservation of protective reflexes, notably the laryngeal reflex. The use of ketamine has been limited because of the occurrence of systemic hypertension in some patients and a high incidence of vivid dreams or hallucinations during recovery; the latter may be prevented by the use of adequate sedative premedication. In addition, movement during operation may be troublesome, particularly in delicate surgery. Nevertheless, in patients with bad facial burns, in other conditions in which the airway is difficult to maintain, and during cardiac catheterization, the drug is useful. A tranquil recovery can be obtained by administration of diazepam before or towards the end of the procedure. Side-effects appear to be less in children, in whom the drug finds its main applications. Because it does not depress the cardiac output, many anaesthetists regard ketamine as the induction agent of choice in the enfeebled patient, and those suffering from hypovolaemic shock or undergoing cardiac surgery.

The drug is administered in a dose range of 1–2 mg/kg by intravenous injection. It can be given by intramuscular injection when the dose is 10 mg/kg. Supplementary injections of ketamine can be used to prolong anaesthesia without the need to give other agents.

Etomidate (Hypnomidate) is a carboxylated imidazole; 0.3 mg/kg is appropriate for the induction of anaesthesia. It is rapidly metabolized and recovery from its effects is rapid and pleasant. Etomidate is thought to be free from the risk of hypersensitivity reactions. It is capable of depressing ventilation but has little adverse effect on the circulation. Disadvantages include pain at the site of injection and occasional but troublesome involuntary muscle movement. Some reports of the drug suggest that it may have a disposition to cause nausea and vomiting during recovery.

The rapid metabolism of etomidate made it seem attractive as a long-term infusion, for example in sedation for intensive care. However, the drug can suppress the secretion of cortisol from the adrenal gland and may have contributed in the past to the death of some severely ill patients. There is no such problem when etomidate is used for induction of anaesthesia.

Benzodiazepines

In recent years there has been a great expansion in the number of benzodiazepine compounds. Table 2.1 gives a summary of the drugs most commonly used in anaesthetic practice. Diazepam, used principally as a tranquillizer, has been given by intravenous injection to induce anaesthesia. It is claimed that it produces less respiratory and circulatory depression than do the barbiturates or propofol. Midazolam (Hypnovel) is a more recent and preferred alternative to diazepam for many circumstances, notably in patients undergoing endoscopic procedures or who are receiving regional anaesthesia (spinal or extradural block, for example). Midazolam may also be used for the induction of anaesthesia in poor risk patients.

One of the features of benzodiazepines is the enormous variability in patient response. In some patients relatively small doses produce the desired level of sedation whereas others are remarkably refractory. Thus in the use of benzodiazepines it is particularly dangerous to have protocols for patient sedation which depend on fixed doses. This comment is particularly important because the administration of these drugs for sedation is not necessarily the specialist activity of the anaesthetist but may be undertaken by practitioners from other disciplines in medicine. Under these circumstances it should be realized that, at high doses in relation to

Table 2.1 Benzodiazepines commonly used in anaesthetic practice

Official name	Tradename	Use	Typical adult dose	Remarks
Diazepam	Valium	oral premedicant	10–20 mg	Variable effect and duration
		i.v. sedation	5–10 mg	Pain, etc., at injection site
Diazepam	Diazemuls	i.v. sedation	5–10 mg	Emulsion. Less pain, etc., than with Valium
Lorazepam	Ativan	oral premedicant i.v. sedation	2–4 mg 1–2 mg	Prolonged amnesia
Temazepam	Normison	oral premedicant	15–30 mg	Faster recovery than with Valium
Midazolam	Hypnovel	i.v. sedation	2.5–7.5 mg	Very rapid recovery
Nitrazepam	Mogadon	oral premedicant hypnotic	5–10 mg	Prolonged hangover effect

patient need, the benzodiazepines can cause respiratory depression or even arrest and the administrator must be skilled in artificial ventilation of the lungs and in other skills in cardiorespiratory support.

Flumazenil is an antagonist to the benzodiazepines. It is not appropriate to use it routinely as a means of reversing the benzodiazepine effect, but is reserved for use in patients who have received a relative overdose of a benzodiazepine. It is worth noting that the duration of flumazenil activity may be shorter than the persisting unwanted effects of the benzodiazepine. Thus the patient should be observed carefully during recovery and supplementary flumazenil may be required. The dose is 1 mg i.v. for an adult.

Neuroleptanalgesia

The drugs used in this technique comprise:

- *Neuroleptic drugs* which produce a state of dissociation—usually a pleasant sensation but sometimes associated with acute anxiety. The best known is dehydrobenzperidol (droperidol). It is a potent anti-emetic agent, depressing the chemoreceptor trigger zone in the midbrain, and has a mild adrenergic blocking effect which is thought by some to protect the peripheral circulation against the 'shock'of surgery. The dose is 5–10 mg i.v. for an average adult. Unfortunately, it may also cause Parkinsonian tremors and delayed feelings of disorientation.
- *Potent analgesics: fentanyl, alfentanil and phenoperidine.* Fentanyl (Sublimaze) is related chemically to pethidine and 0.1 mg is approximately equipotent with morphine 10 mg. The duration of analgesia with fentanyl is about 20–40 minutes. It shares with pethidine the ability to produce nausea and vomiting, cardiorespiratory depression and, in the long term, addiction. Phenoperidine (Operidine) has pharmacological effects which are very similar to those of fentanyl except that the duration of analgesia of 2 mg of the drug ($\doteqdot$ 10 mg of morphine) is about 90 minutes.

Mixtures of fentanyl with droperidol (Thalamonal) may be used to induce a state of unconsciousness with profound analgesia. Anaesthesia is maintained, thereafter, with nitrous oxide and oxygen and, when required, with a muscle relaxant drug. While it is claimed that a stable arterial pressure and some protection from shock is provided by the neuroleptanalgesic combination of drugs, it is the opinion of many that, apart from the duration of action of fentanyl and phenoperidine, the advantage of neuroleptanalgesia over the use of the more traditional analgesics, such as morphine, in the maintenance of anaesthesia is not striking.

Sufentanyl has characteristics similar to fentanyl but is less likely to cause the level of bradycardia that sometimes accompanies fentanyl. The dose of sufentanyl is 5–10 mcg/kg. It has become popular as a component in total intravenous anaesthesia.

Alfentanil has a shorter duration of action than fentanyl; it is especially suited to techniques for maintaining anaesthesia by the intravenous route in combination with drugs such as propofol or etomidate, for day-case anaesthesia in which a relatively rapid recovery from the effect of the opioid is particularly important. The dose for an adult is in the range of 5–10 mcg/kg.

DRUGS USED FOR PREMEDICATION

Premedication is a general term describing the administration of drugs given before anaesthesia to facilitate the process of anaesthesia and for postoperative care. The principal reasons for premedication are to:

- relieve anxiety
- reduce pain
- contribute to the effect produced by general anaesthetics during the operation (reducing MAC requirement)
- abolish or reduce undesirable parasympathetic activity
- reduce postoperative nausea and vomiting
- reduce acidity and volume of gastric contents in circumstances in which regurgitation of gastric contents is particularly likely.

Apart from the last of these reasons administration of premedicant drugs is much less common than in the past. Changing attitudes to hospitals and disease are considered by many to have reduced the level of anxiety in many patients before operation. The need for pain relief remains in some surgical emergencies, but the contribution of analgesics to the general anaesthetic effect or to the level of analgesia in the postoperative period can be achieved in many circumstances by the administration of appropriate opioids at the beginning of or during the operation.

The need for minimizing parasympathetic activity was most obvious in the days when diethyl ether was used because it resulted in frightening stimulation of oropharyngeal secretions. Routine administration of anticholinergics to block parasympathetic activity can be unpleasant for the patient before operation because dryness of the mouth can be extreme. If there is a need for parasympathetic blockade during anaesthesia, for example if the heart rate becomes undesirably slow, the anaesthetist can give an anticholinergic intravenously at that time.

The relief of anxiety (sedation)

When pain is present acutely before operation, anxiety may be relieved by alleviating pain. In most cases, however, reassurance and simple explanation to the patient can save much in the way of drugs. Patients will benefit from a simple explanation of hospital routine as it affects the events of which they will be aware before and after the operation (transport to the operating room, preparations for monitoring, etc.). A careful preoperative visit by the members of the operating team, particularly the anaesthetist, is invaluable. Clear explanations should be given of all aspects of management during which the patient will be aware or expected to cooperate. The use of nerve block without general anaesthesia is a particularly good example.

If drugs are to be used to produce sedation and analgesia, morphine remains the opiate of choice unless the patient cannot tolerate morphine because of nausea or vomiting. Papaveretum is a mixture of the alkaloids of opium and, if available, may produce less nausea and vomiting than does morphine.

Pethidine hydrochloride was originally introduced as a substitute for morphine. Compared with morphine it is a poorer sedative and produces less euphoria.

Benzodiazepines. These have specific anti-anxiety properties and can be given orally, which is very welcome in nursing routines. Of the drugs listed in Table 2.1 temazepam is by far the most popular. Given in a dose of 15–30 mg orally not more than 2 hours before operation it can induce a very acceptable degree of calmness with a mild feeling of drowsiness. In many patients, the effect of temazepam although real is hardly able to be recognized by the casual onlooker; the patient, however, appears to be calm and rational.

Phenothiazines. Some drugs of this class can produce acceptable anxiolysis and sedation before operation. The principal example in current practice is the use of trimeprazine syrup (Vallergan)

2–4 mg/kg given orally to children. Some of the phenothiazines have important anti-emetic effects and cyclizine may be used particularly in the postoperative period. When administered with opiates it reduces the risk of nausea and vomiting significantly.

Anticholinergics. There are three compounds of importance: atropine, glycopyrrolate and hyoscine. All minimize parasympathetic overactivity. Hyoscine causes a variable degree of sedation and has an anti-emetic effect. Neither of these actions occurs in the case of the other two drugs. Marked dilatation of the pupil may occur, particularly with atropine which also may produce a mild degree of cerebral stimulation. Glycopyrrolate, which does not cross the blood–brain barrier, is free of this effect on the brain.

NEUROMUSCULAR BLOCKING DRUGS

Tubocurarine (curare), introduced in 1942, was the earliest drug to be used as a muscle relaxant in anaesthesia. Nowadays there are many drugs to choose from and in comparing their value the anaesthetic will have special regard to the following factors:

The type of block. The majority of drugs act by competing with acetylcholine at both pre- and postjunctional receptors (Fig. 2.3). The receptor affinities of different myoneural blockers vary.

Duration of action. A fast onset of effect may be important when there is a need for rapid tracheal intubation to secure the airway. A prolonged recovery is inappropriate if the drug is used for a short operation. Above all, however, predictability of speed of onset and time of recovery are important.

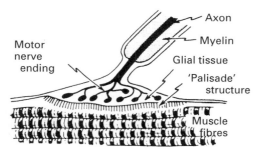

Fig. 2.3   The myoneural junction: the palisade structure is the site at which acetylcholine, released from the motor nerve endings, acts upon the muscle fibres to cause contraction.

Method of excretion or detoxication in the body. Failure of renal or hepatic function respectively can lead to prolongation of action. Pipecuronium, for example, is largely dependent on renal excretion. Atracurium undergoes spontaneous breakdown of the molecule (Hofmann degradation) and this is especially useful in organ failure.

Ease of antagonism of the block following the administration of an anticholinesterase drug such as neostigmine.

Possibility of histamine release following injection.

Side-effects. Muscle relaxant drugs may mimic or block the effects of acetylcholine on other cholinergic receptors. Thus they may produce ganglion blockade or parasympathomimetic effects.

Compatibility with other drugs which may be given in the course of anaesthesia, including synergism and antagonism of the effects of either drug.

It must be stressed that the muscle relaxants have no analgesic or anaesthetic properties. It is essential therefore that the patient receives additional drugs to ensure analgesia and anaesthesia. Ventilation must be maintained by artificial means.

PHARMACOLOGY OF MUSCLE RELAXANT AGENTS

Competitive or non-depolarizing relaxants

Tubocurarine. The South-American Indians used curare as an arrow poison; their victims were paralysed and died from asphyxia. The drug is still refined from the extracts of plants brought from South America. Its principal interest nowadays is historic since it was the first muscle relaxant used in anaesthesia. The dose for the average adult is about 30 mg i.v. Paralysis of muscles, including the respiratory muscles, develops within about 3 minutes and adequate time must be allowed for the drug to act. There is a moderate reduction in arterial pressure, due in part to histamine release. With larger doses ganglion blockade may occur resulting in more marked reduction in arterial pressure. The effect of tubocurarine lasts from 30 to 40 minutes as a rough approximation.

Alcuronium (Alloferin) is about twice as potent as tubocurarine but has otherwise similar properties, although it is less likely to release histamine from the tissues. The dose is 0.15–0.25 mg/kg. The duration of effect is about 25 minutes.

Pancuronium bromide (Pavulon) is five to six times more potent than tubocurarine. It has little effect on the circulation, although mild hypertension and tachycardia have been reported occasionally. The dose is 0.07 mg/kg and the duration of action is about 45 minutes. Even a small overdose of pancuronium will cause profound block which may be refractory to attempted antagonism with neostigmine. The drug is excreted in the urine, but a significant proportion is metabolized in the liver.

Atracurium (Tracrium) is chemically related to tubocurarine. The recommended dose is 0.3 mg/kg. Atracurium is claimed to be almost devoid of any influence on the cardiovascular system, although in some patients there may be histamine release. It is effectively broken down in the bloodstream either by the influence of cholinesterase or by a spontaneous breakdown process known as Hofmann elimination. The drug is noted for the speed of onset of blockade, which is usually sufficient to allow tracheal intubation within 90 seconds of injection. The duration of action of an average dose is about 30 minutes. It is usually necessary to administer an anticholinesterase such as neostigmine to antagonize the block. The pattern of metabolism of atracurium makes it particularly suitable as a neuromuscular blocking drug for patients with renal failure.

Vecuronium (Norcuron) is similar to atracurium in respect of its lack of effect on the cardiovascular system and the rapidity of onset and recovery of the block. The duration of the block following an average dose (0.1 mg/kg) is about 30 minutes. Vecuronium is partly metabolized in the liver and small amounts may be excreted in the urine, but the metabolic fate of the drug is not known in detail. It may be less suited than atracurium for patients with renal failure but, in contrast, it is not thought likely to cause histamine release.

Both atracurium and vecuronium may be particularly suited to continuous infusion regimens, a method not previously considered seriously for the administration of neuromuscular blocking drugs. Both have gained greatly in popularity since their introduction. Even when given as a single injection the rapid onset of effect and the good quality of recovery, compared with earlier drugs, are seen as a great advantage.

Pipecuronium (Arduan) is structurally related to pancuronium. It has a relatively slow onset of action and a long duration of 90 minutes.

Doxicurium, which is not yet available for clinical use in the UK, also has a slow onset and has a duration of about 60 minutes.

Mivacurium (Mivacron) is a short acting drug with an onset of effect suitable for tracheal intubation within 2 minutes. The duration of action is 10–20 minutes. At the time of writing it is enjoying some success in anaesthesia for day-case surgery.

Rocuronium. This compound was developed at the same laboratories as vecuronium. It has a slightly more rapid onset of effect than vecuronium with the same duration of action. The dose for an average adult is likely to be in the range 40–50 mg, although it must be noted that the clinical evaluation of this compound is not complete at the time of writing.

Antagonism of the non-depolarizing relaxants

Neostigmine (Prostigmin), which is an anticholinesterase, allows the concentration of acetylcholine to increase and is an antagonist to the non-depolarizing muscle relaxants. The dose of neostigmine is typically 2.5–5 mg. i.v. for an adult.

Suxamethonium

Suxamethonium chloride (Scoline, Anectine) has an action similar to that of acetylcholine. There is initial muscle twitching and fasciculation followed by paralysis which last from 2 to 4 minutes following a dose of 0.6–1.2 mg/kg. There is a transient increase in arterial pressure and often a slowing of heart rate which may be particularly marked following a second or subsequent injection of suxamethonium. This effect can be minimized by the intravenous administration of atropine. Suxamethonium can produce a transient small increase in sodium potassium concentration. This is of little importance in normal subjects but can cause dangerous cardiac arrhythmia if there is pre-existing hyperkalaemia such as may be associated with gross tissue damage in tissue crushing injuries or burns. Suxamethonium is hydrolyzed in the blood by pseudocholinesterase found in the plasma. In some cases this enzyme might be atypical or may be abnormally low in concentration and the effect of suxamethonium on neuromuscular blockade may be prolonged for a considerable period. There is no antagonist to this effect although benefit may come from giving fresh frozen plasma which contains pseudocholinesterase. Under most circumstances, however, the lungs should be ventilated artificially until spontaneous recovery occurs. Even in the presence of high concentrations of abnormal enzymes, apnoea is unlikely to exceed 8 hours.

ARE ANAESTHETICS TERATOGENIC?

It can be shown that in the course of a day's work in an operating theatre the staff acquire measurable trace concentrations of anaesthetics in the blood and other tissues, and there is concern that these may be teratogenic. Experimental studies in small animals suggest that chronic exposure to some of the inhalation anaesthetics can induce a variety of abnormalities, the most consistent being an influence on a developing fetus: a reduction in litter weight and size, resorption of the embryo (a process analogous to spontaneous abortion) and congenital abnormality of offspring.

Controlled epidemiological studies have suggested that pregnant theatre staff may be at risk from similar mechanisms, although the true significance of such observations is controversial. Nevertheless it is accepted that staff should avoid unnecessary exposure to anaesthetic gases and, in the UK, there is official advice on the use of ducting (scavenging) systems to vent the patient's expired gas to the outside environment. For the same reasons women who are, or who are likely to be, pregnant should not receive any general (or local) anaesthetic drug during the first trimester unless they are to undergo surgery for a life-threatening condition such as acute appendicitis.

3. Anaesthetic machines and apparatus

The anaesthetic 'machine' is composed of five simple systems (Fig. 3.1):

- a supply of compressed gas at a pressure of 413 kPa
- a method of controlling the release of gas from the high pressure system
- a method of metering the gases
- a method of vaporizing volatile anaesthetic agents
- a means of delivering the gases and vapours to the patient.

Different manufacturers design their anaesthetic machines in different ways, all working to achieve a compact, user-friendly and, above all, safe system for inhalation anaesthesia. In addition to the basic components listed, there are various safety devices to warn of failure of delivery of the intended mixture to be inhaled. A work surface is usually incorporated and many systems include an automatic lung ventilator.

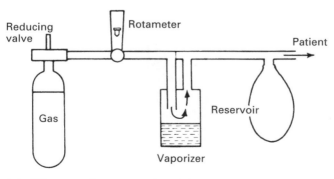

Fig. 3.1 Diagrammatic representation of the five components of a simple anaesthetic apparatus.

The supply of gases

This may take one of two forms. In most hospitals oxygen and nitrous oxide are each delivered by a supply pipe from a central source. There are reserve cylinders of oxygen and nitrous oxide on each anaesthetic machine trolley in case the central supply should fail. In some, increasingly rare, situations in modern hospitals and in some hospitals where there is less sophistication nitrous oxide and oxygen may come exclusively from cylinders mounted on the trolley. The cylinders are readily identifiable, each being painted in a distinctive colour:

oxygen	—	black with white shoulders
nitrous oxide	—	blue

In addition, the name of the gas is printed on the cylinder, as is the chemical symbol. As a safeguard against connecting a cylinder to the wrong inlet or valve the head of the cylinder, beside the part from which the gas flows, has two small holes drilled in positions specific for each gas (Fig. 3.2). These match two pins on the

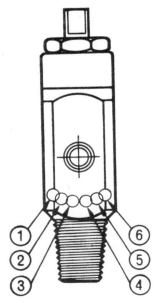

Fig. 3.2   This diagram shows how the holes on the cylinder neck are drilled on an arc. Only two holes are found on each cylinder, e.g.: 2 and 5 on oxygen cylinders, 3 and 5 on nitrous oxide cylinders.

appropriate yoke or inlet usually leading to the reducing valve or pressure regulator (see Fig. 3.3).

It is important to know how much gas each cylinder contains. In the cases of oxygen, the reducing valve connected to the cylinder has attached to it a pressure gauge and the contents of the cylinder can be estimated by noting the pressure. A full cylinder contains gas at a pressure of approximately 13.8×10^6 Pa and as the volume of gas in the cylinder decreases the pressure is reduced proportionately. Nitrous oxide is stored as a liquid and consequently the pressure of the gas above the liquid does not change in a linear manner as the cylinder empties until approximately one-third of the contents remains. With fuller cylinders there will be some reduction in pressure during use which reflects a decrease in cylinder temperature as liquid nitrous oxide is converted to gas (latent heat of vaporization). Finally, the contents of a nitrous oxide cylinder can be ascertained by weighing the cylinder and subtracting the tare weight which is embossed on the neck (100 litres of liquid nitrous oxide weigh 0.8 kg).

Reducing valves or pressure regulators

Pipeline supply systems, which are coloured (Table 3.1) blue or white on the outside depending on the gas conveyed, deliver from the central source at a pressure of 413 kPa. This pressure is appropriate for metering the gases and is a power supply for some types of equipment, such as suction or lung ventilators. Pressures of the gases in cylinders vary from 48.3×10^5 to 13.8×10^6 Pa. Such high pressures are not easily manageable and they must be **reduced** to workable levels. A pressure regulating valve is used for this purpose (Fig. 3.3). They are built onto the anaesthetic machine (Fig. 3.4).

Table 3.1   Colour codes in gas conducting systems

Gas	Cylinder	Pipeline
Oxygen	Black/white shoulder	White
Nitrous oxide	Blue	Blue
N_2O/O_2	Blue/white shoulder	Blue/white
Air	Grey/white & black shoulder	White/black
Vacuum		Yellow

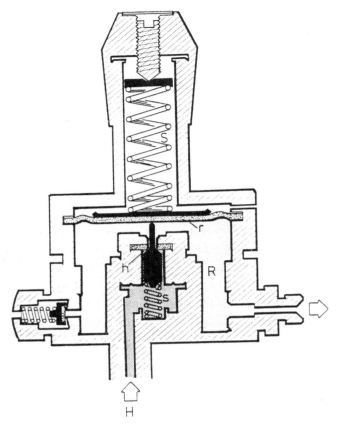

Fig. 3.3 Working principle of a pressure regulator. The high pressure gas from the cylinder enters the system at H and gas at the reduced pressure leaves the port shown on the bottom right of the drawing. The value of the reduced pressure (R) is set by the force applied from S (upper) to the diaphragm (r). As gas escapes from the system when in use there is a tendency for r to descend pushing the dense black valve device downwards against s and opening h. This allows the pressure R to be maintained. The valve device in the bottom left-hand part of the drawing allows escape of gas to atmosphere should pressure R become excessive for any unexpected reason.

Flow meters

Flow meters on anaesthetic machines are commonly, and sometimes incorrectly, known as Rotameters (the trade name of the largest manufacturer of these instruments). They consist of tapered glass tubes in which an aluminium bobbin spins (Fig. 3.5).

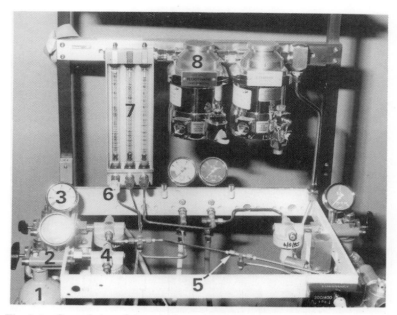

Fig. 3.4 General view of anaesthetic machine with top working surface removed to show, particularly, the pressure regulators and gas conducting pipes. 1: oxygen cylinder (black with white collar); 2: pin index mounting; 3: pressure gauge; 4: pressure regulator; 5: gas conducting pipe, this particular one connecting from the oxygen supply to the emergency oxygen outlet; 6: flow meter control (turn anti-clockwise to open); 7: flow meter bank; 8: temperature-compensated vaporizer for halothane or Fluothane.

The gas flow is indicated by the height of the top part of the bobbin and is read against the scale marked on the tube.

Vaporizers

Although it is little used nowadays, an old-style vaporizer for volatile anaesthetics is shown in Figure 3.6; the exact concentration of vapour emitted sometimes varies with the duration of use on any one day and is not regarded as critical. A lever at the side of the bottle directs an increasing amount of the gas into the bottle and when the plunger is depressed the stream of gas coming from the 'J' tube is directed on to or through the fluid in the bottle.

Many factors govern the concentration of volatile anaesthetic given off from this simple vaporizer. Among these are:

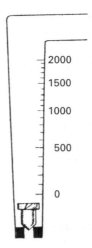

Fig. 3.5   Flow meter. As gas enters at the lower end, the spinning bobbin rises in proportion to the flow of gas.

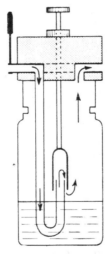

Fig. 3.6   A simple vaporizer, the Boyle's bottle. Arrows indicate the direction of gas flow.

- ambient pressure and temperature
- temperature and vapour pressure of the agent
- rate of carrier gas flow through the vaporizer
- area of the gas/liquid interface
- position and movement of the vaporizer.

The commonest vaporizer used in the UK (Fig. 3.4) compensates automatically for changes in the factors mentioned above and can deliver known concentrations of vapour for which it has been designed, usually in increments of 0.5%. Each vaporizer is designed for a specific volatile anaesthetic (halothane, enflurane or isoflurane). These vaporizers should never be filled with anything other than the liquid for which they have been designed and calibrated. Because of the vaporizing characteristics of desflurane the design of its vaporizer is radically different from the example shown in Figure 3.4. Desflurane vaporizers incorporate an electrical supply which facilitates heating and therefore vaporization of the liquid.

Delivery of gases and vapours to the patient

The Magill attachment (Fig. 3.7) consists of a corrugated rubber or plastic tube, a reservoir bag and a spill valve. The reservoir is necessary since the flow of gas from the machine is continuous during all phases of breathing whereas the patient's demands for these gases occur only during inspiration. At the patient's end of the tube is placed the unidirectional spill valve (Heidbrink) through which excess gas may pass during expiration. The immediate connection to the patient is made with a mask, which is placed over the patient's face, or with a laryngeal mask or a tracheal tube. When using this type of breathing system (sometimes loosely called 'circuit'), it is necessary to deliver from the machine a flow of gases at least equal to the patient's alveolar minute volume (usually 5–6 litres/minute are given), otherwise carbon dioxide will accumulate and will be rebreathed. The system should not

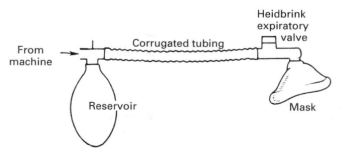

Fig. 3.7   Magill attachment.

be used for more than a few minutes if ventilation of the lungs is controlled artificially.

A non-return and non-rebreathing valve (Fig. 3.8) may be used instead of the conventional Heidbrink valve. In this case, during expiration all the expired gas passes to the atmosphere and rebreathing of carbon dioxide is minimal.

The T-piece system (Fig. 3.9) introduced by Ayre is especially useful in children when the resistance to expiration offered by valves is harmful to the child, particularly if spontaneous breathing is to occur for a prolonged period. The open limb of the T-piece conveys expired gas to the atmosphere and acts as a reservoir.

A coaxial system has two tubes, one inside the other. There are two examples: the Bain system (Fig. 3.10A) and the Lack system (Fig. 3.10B). The former is similar in function to a T-piece except that there is a spill valve and a reservoir bag on the expiratory limb. The Lack system is similar to the Magill system except that the spill valve is placed away from the patient end of the system, the inner tube acting as a conduit to it.

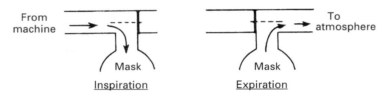

Fig. 3.8   Non-return valve. During inspiration the valve slides across and permits the patient to breathe gases from the machine. On expiration the valve cuts off the supply of gases from the machine and allows the gas expired by the patient to pass to the atmosphere.

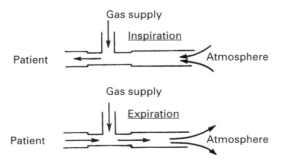

Fig. 3.9   T-piece principle. As there are no valves, resistance is minimal and, by adjusting the flow of gases and the length of the expiratory limb to the atmosphere, the degree of rebreathing can be controlled.

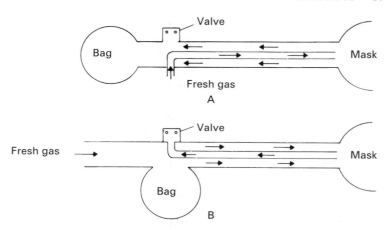

Fig. 3.10   A. Bain coaxial system. B. Lack coaxial system.

The main purpose of these systems is to allow what appears to be one tube between the machine and the patient. They allow the spill valve, which may need to be adjusted from time to time with a scavenging shroud placed over it (see below), to be well clear of the patient's head. This is particularly important in head and neck operations when access to the region around the head may become difficult.

Total and partial rebreathing: the circle system (Fig. 3.11)

The patient's expired gas passes in the expiratory limb of a circle through soda lime (a mixture of calcium hydroxide 95% and sodium hydroxide 5%) which absorbs carbon dioxide almost completely. The gas then passes to the reservoir bag and can be used again. In a *closed* circuit system the fresh gas supply is limited to the replacement of net losses to the patient: anaesthetics taken up and oxygen required for metabolism, the latter amounting to 250 ml/min or less. Most often these systems are used with more than the minimum fresh gas flow described above: perhaps 1–3 litres/min of a mixture of oxygen, nitrous oxide and a volatile agent such as enflurane. A rebreathing system offers several advantages:

- economy of gases and vapours
- conservation of moisture and heat
- less contamination of the environment with anaesthetic gases.

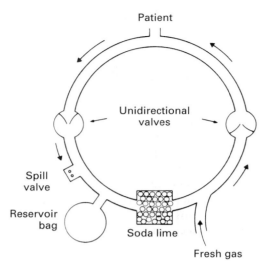

Fig. 3.11 Circle CO_2 absorption system.

The amount of rubber or plastic tubing required, the valves, which must be interposed to keep the gases flowing in the correct direction, and soda lime all add resistance to spontaneous breathing. During controlled ventilation the increase in resistance to gas flow is of no importance since the work of breathing is undertaken by a lung ventilator or by the anaesthetist squeezing the reservoir bag. The increased resistance to breathing in a circle system, however, is usually unacceptable for children.

Total and partial rebreathing systems have been relatively unpopular in western Europe in the past, although always popular in the USA. Certainly part of the reluctance in the UK was uncertainty in knowing accurately the concentration of gases and vapours delivered to the patient. The advent of inexpensive and reliable gas analysers and of new, more expensive, volatile agents such as desflurane have given a new impetus to rebreathing systems.

Scavenging of anaesthetic gases

In all the breathing systems mentioned so far arrangements are made to capture gases and vapours escaping from the exhaust valve or flow outlet so that they can be conducted to the environment outside of the hospital building. This is a safeguard of the health of operating theatre personnel. There are two scavenging methods in common use:

Passive removal. The gases are led outside the hospital building via a metal conduit. The flow along the conduit is caused by the patient's expiratory effort. This method is simple and inexpensive but care must be taken to ensure that the resistance of flow is not excessive and that condensed water vapour does not accumulate in the conduit with a risk of retrograde flow in the direction of the patient.

Active removal. This is the commonest form in modern hospitals. The gases are led to a reservoir on the anaesthetic trolley from which a pump carries them through narrow-bore tubing to the outside of the building. Such systems are expensive to install but are safer than passive systems and are essential if the operating suite is situated at some distance from the outside walls of the building.

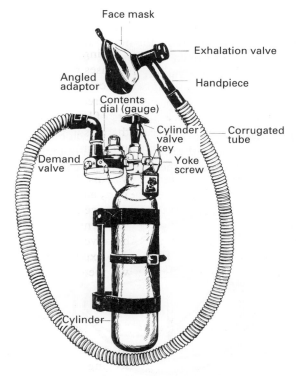

Fig. 3.12   Entonox apparatus for self-administered 50% nitrous oxide in oxygen. The gas leaves the cylinder only when the patient makes an inspiratory effort.

Intermittent flow machines

Most anaesthetic machines are based on the continuous flow principle; that is, the fresh gas flows to the circuit at a constant rate throughout all phases of breathing, the excess during expiration being accommodated in a reservoir. Other systems such as the Entonox (premixed 50% nitrous oxide in oxygen) analgesia apparatus supply gases to a patient only in response to the patient's inspiratory effort (Fig. 3.12). In using a system of this type it is essential to ensure a gas-tight fit between the patient's face and the mask or the system will not function satisfactorily.

Aficionados of very old movies may have seen the hero or heroine overcome almost instantly by a state of anaesthesia induced by the villain who has applied an anaesthetic soaked handkerchief to the subject's nose and mouth. All anaesthetists are impressed by the speed with which it happens. Although the earliest forms of inhalation anaesthesia were similar in principle, it took longer to achieve the desired effect. The Schimmelbusch mask (Fig. 3.13) was originally introduced for use with chloroform; although mainly of historic interest, it represents the next stage up in sophistication. The frame which held linen was applied loosely to the nose and mouth and the carrier gas was air.

Draw-over vaporizers

While open masks such as the Schimmelbusch have the advantage of portability, many of the disadvantages—notably variability in the concentration of anaesthetic inspired—can be overcome by

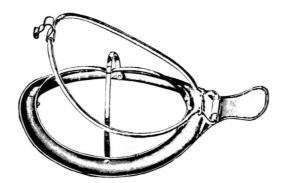

Fig. 3.13   Schimmelbusch's mask.

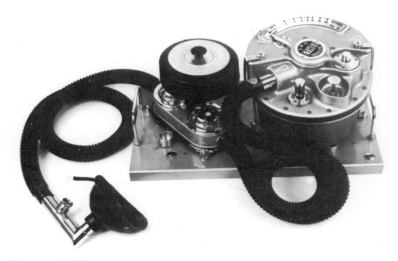

Fig. 3.14 EMO apparatus.

using the EMO temperature compensated ether draw-over vaporizer (Fig. 3.14). The patient inhales atmospheric air through the
vaporizing chamber, and the design ensures that the inspired concentration of ether is known accurately. The bellows system,
shown on the centre of the figure, acts as a reservoir and also as a
method of monitoring breathing. If the anaesthetist wishes to ventilate the lungs artificially, manual compression of the bellows provides a source of gas under positive pressure. The system can be
used to control ventilation in a patient who has received a neuromuscular blocking drug; 3–4% of ether in air will be sufficient to
provide an anaesthetizing gas mixture under these circumstances.

Where there is a need to enrich the oxygen content of the
inspired gas, oxygen from a cylinder can be admitted through a
port incorporated in the bellows system. It should be remembered,
of course, that ether in oxygen-rich air is explosive. The EMO system is still of great service in producing anaesthesia for surgical
operations in the developing world.

4. Pre-anaesthetic examination and therapy

It is important that all doctors and nurses, irrespective of their practice discipline, know the problems and difficulties that may arise from unrecognized disease in patients presenting for anaesthesia and operation. Although all patients should be seen by the anaesthetist before anaesthesia this may not be feasible until perhaps the night before or day of operation. In the past attempts have been made to organize special anaesthetic outpatient clinics so that patients may be seen several days or even weeks before operation but this is often impractical and it is expensive of medical manpower. It also has to be recognized that the patterns of flow to elective operating lists are changing. In some circumstances general practitioners or family doctors have direct access to certain operating lists. In other situations the practice of day-case surgery is blossoming and in these circumstances the person who is first in contact with the patient at the clinic, usually a surgeon, should understand the difference between normal and abnormal conditions in respect of anaesthesia, the criteria for entry to an outpatient list, and recognize the patient who should be admitted for a more detailed preoperative workup.

PRE-ANAESTHETIC EXAMINATION

History

Special attention is paid to the history of previous anaesthetics, particularly if the patient or the notes reveal a complication that is likely to recur. Anaphylactoid reactions come under this heading, and sensitivities to antibacterial agents, skin preparations and skin dressings are quite common. Rarer conditions range from suxamethonium apnoea (p. 37), malignant hyperpyrexia (p. 130) to delay in recovery from anaesthesia, which may accompany

53

hypothyroidism. These are examples rather than an exhaustive list. The patient's mode of life, occupation, and habits regarding exercise, alcohol and tobacco may all be pointers to the general state of health. It is useful to ask if any close blood relatives have experienced any problems or complications when undergoing anaesthesia as there are sometimes genetic factors in adverse reactions to drugs. Note the personal preferences of each patient for individual techniques. A special note should be made of anaesthetics administered within the previous 6 months because the anaesthetist may wish to avoid repeated exposure to halothane.

While taking the history, the anaesthetist has an opportunity to assess the patient's nervous temperament and this will give some guide to prescribing preoperative sedation.

Surgical condition for which the operation is proposed. Elicit any symptoms or signs which may be relevant to the anaesthetic; for example, a patient who has been bleeding may be anaemic.

Symptoms suggestive of cardiorespiratory insufficiency or disease. Questions are directed to symptoms such as cough, breathlessness on exertion, episodes of chest pain and swelling of the ankles.

While the patient's history regarding cough, breathlessness on exertion and his degree of exercise tolerance are of considerable importance in assessing fitness for anaesthesia, routine clinical examination is equally important. Chest radiography should be performed in all patients undergoing major surgery. Apart from being a useful screen for preoperative disease the X-ray allows comparison in the event of postoperative abnormalities. Where the history or examination indicates limitation of function or of exercise tolerance, special respiratory function tests may be carried out. These are discussed below (p. 58). The haemoglobin concentration should be measured. Although there is some variation in what is considered an acceptable haemoglobin concentration for elective surgery, it should normally be greater than 10g/dl.

Sickle-cell disease, and even sickle-cell trait, pose risks if the patient becomes hypoxaemic for any reason. The Sickledex test is a useful primary screen.

Urinary system

The urine is examined chemically and microscopically for any abnormal constituents such as sugar, albumen, blood or cells. Where any of these is present, further investigation of the urinary tract is undertaken. In many cases, particularly those patients undergoing major surgery, the blood urea concentration is measured.

Nutrition and hydration

In most patients admitted for elective surgery, little abnormality will be noted in this respect, but in patients who have been suffering from wasting diseases or who have been vomiting or losing fluids from fistulae, it is important that blood should be sent for measurement of the plasma proteins and electrolytes, liver function tests and acid–base indices.

The system to be operated on should be examined if this is likely to have a particular bearing on the anaesthetic.

The nose, throat and teeth should be examined carefully for signs of deformity or infection which may influence the maintenance of an airway. Particular note should be made of any special dental features such as loose teeth, crowns, etc. The superficial veins should be examined carefully. Where it is intended to use a regional analgesic technique, the area of the proposed injection should be examined to ensure that there are no signs of local infection in the skin.

Drug history

Details should be sought of any drugs which the patient is taking or has taken during the recent past. In all cases the anaesthetist should consider any likely drug interactions which might occur in the course of surgery. Common examples include antihypertensive agents (beta-blockers, calcium channel blockers and ACE inhibitors). These drugs should not be discontinued during the course of surgery and anaesthesia but anaesthetic administration should be cautious because of an enhanced risk of a reduced cardiac output. The vast majority of patients are capable of continuing medication, where appropriate, although the general anaesthetic management would normally prescribe that 'nothing should be taken by mouth'. Patients receiving digoxin should continue therapy and those with a history of angina may benefit from the application of a glyceryl trinitrate patch, or transdermal administration, before anaesthesia commences. Those who are in the habit of using bronchodilator aerosols should continue to do so in the pre- and postoperative periods.

Oral contraceptives may inhibit the liver microsomal enzymes.

Pethidine, for example, may be metabolized more slowly in these circumstances. Oestrogen-containing oral contraceptives may increase the incidence of venous thrombosis during and after operation, and some authorities believe that it is better to stop these drugs 4 weeks before surgery if possible. Otherwise, or perhaps in any case, subcutaneous heparin 5000 units should be given to reduce the risk of thrombosis. Progesterone contraceptives are comparatively safe. Patients receiving hormone replacement-therapy should not discontinue their medication.

Where examination reveals alteration in the serum electrolyte concentrations, intravenous therapy should be commenced to ensure that these deficiencies are remedied before anaesthesia and operation.

Patients with a history of skeletal disease present a variety of problems. These include the need for special care in moving the patient, particularly during periods of unconsciousness, and limited neck and jaw movements which may indicate difficulty in airway management including laryngoscopy. Inability to move the spine normally can compromise attempts to achieve spinal or epidural block.

Patients with hepatocellular and renal disease may respond adversely to a variety of drugs which depend on these organs for metabolism and excretion.

RESPIRATORY DISEASE

In the acute phases of a common cold elective anaesthesia is not advised. Modification of ciliary activity, inability to cough effectively in some cases, and complete or partial blockage of the upper airway are all obvious difficulties.

The assessment of chronic lung disease calls for careful preoperative study and planning. Patients with airways narrowing (e.g. asthma) must be managed with appropriate bronchodilator therapy to achieve the optimal conditions. Often the patient is the best judge as to when that has occurred. Patients with restrictive lung disease have a limited vital capacity and a greater potential risk of postoperative ventilatory failure, particularly when the operation has been performed in the abdomen or chest. The presence of copious purulent secretions, for example bronchiectasis, may indicate a period of lung physiotherapy and antibiotics. Even then special arrangements may have to be instituted to facilitate effective expectoration in the postoperative period, including perhaps a decision to use an extradural block for postoperative pain relief.

The significance of pulmonary disease in a patient awaiting

anaesthesia and operation is not connected with the fact that the anaesthetist may use the lungs as a route of administration of drugs; although the uptake of the inhalation anaesthetics may be impaired, for example in the patient with chronic bronchitis, the problem is not insuperable. The real difficulty relates to the *reserves* of lung function and whether or not these will be sufficient to allow the patient to withstand the physiological impairment, which is a consequence of the operation, so that adequate lung function can be ensured in the postoperative period. The following considerations apply:

- Where neuromuscular blocking drugs have been used, there is inevitably a small impairment of ventilatory capacity for several hours after operation. A patient with diminished ventilatory capacity, as a result of disease, may be at risk from developing postoperative ventilatory failure if the danger is not recognized and appropriate monitoring is not instituted.
- As explained on page 23, there is an increase in right-to-left shunting of blood within the lungs as a consequence of anaesthesia, and the effects of abdominal surgery may aggravate this effect. For example, the patient who has undergone upper abdominal surgery can be expected to have a reduction of the arterial Po_2 of 3–4 kPa in the postoperative period (breathing air). This reduction will continue for 2–3 days after operation. This effect is a consequence of the anaesthetic initially, but wound pain, pneumoperitoneum and distension of bowel are the principal factors beyond the first 2 hours after surgery. These surgical factors may diminish the ventilatory capacity also.

Excessive production of secretions by the bronchial mucosa may cause additional respiratory embarrassment to the patient who is unable to expectorate as a consequence of pain or debility, or both. Retained secretions will lead eventually to absorption collapse of segments of the lung.

Most of the important clues are to be found in the history. Questioning should be directed to the frequency and extent of previous illness related to the lungs, with special reference to the need for antibiotic therapy and admission to hospital. The occurrence of breathlessness is an estimate of the patient's tolerance of exercise and should be noted. The quantity of sputum production and the quality and colour of the expectorate are important, as is the patient's smoking habit. Even in the absence of a history of pulmonary disease, the heavy smoker can be expected to have an abnormally high sputum production.

The clinical examination of the chest will reveal signs of localized lung disease and the general signs of chronic bronchitis and emphysema in the more severe cases, but it is worth remembering that a patient with seriously limited lung function may exhibit few abnormal signs on percussion and auscultation of the chest and that the important pointers are to be found in the history. The presence of finger clubbing is a valuable sign of intrapulmonary sepsis. Special attention should be paid to the configuration of the chest; for example, the presence of marked kyphoscoliosis is almost invariably associated with diminished ventilatory function and chronic inflammatory changes in the lung tissue.

On X-ray, evidence of fibrosis and emphysema of the lung fields may be obvious, but often abnormal changes, if any, are non-specific.

As a general rule, all patients undergoing abdominal surgery, with or without symptoms referable to the lungs, and all patients with a history of pulmonary disease should be X-rayed before anaesthesia and operation. Apart from a possible role in evaluation, the preoperative chest X-ray provides a baseline in the event of respiratory problems in the postoperative period.

Lung function tests

Arterial blood should be sampled for the estimation of Po_2, Pco_2 and pH. Where there is pre-existing hypoxaemia (Po_2, less than 8 kPa, breathing air), and the patient is about to undergo abdominal surgery, it is unlikely that adequate oxygenation can be maintained in the postoperative period without artificial ventilation for 1–2 days and oxygen enrichment of the inspired gas.

If there is carbon dioxide retention (Pco_2, more than 6 kPa) before operation, it should be appreciated that the patient is likely to depend on the 'hypoxic drive' to ventilation and that excessive enrichment of the inspired oxygen concentration during spontaneous breathing may, paradoxically, aggravate ventilatory depression. In such patients it may be desirable to institute positive pressure ventilation both during the operation and, if necessary, in the postoperative period.

Although there is a wide range of spirometric tests, few of these are of much value in preoperative assessment. One exception is the measurement of the vital capacity and the forced vital capacity (FVC) using a spirometer such as the Vitalograph (Fig. 4.1). The patient exhales to the spirometer at a rate of his choice until no

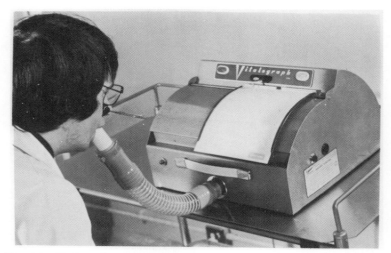

Fig. 4.1 Vitalograph apparatus in use.

more gas can be expelled from the lungs (vital capacity). The forced vital capacity is the same manoeuvre undertaken in the minimum period of time. In the case of an adult of average size, the vital capacity should be in the range of 3–5.5 litres. The effect of upper abdominal surgery will reduce this by about 55% in the first 2 days after operation. Patients with restrictive lung disease will suffer the same percentage impairment so that if the preoperative vital capacity is only 900 ml, they must undertake a maximum ventilatory effort to achieve a tidal volume of 400–450 ml. Not only is this exhausting for the patient, but any further reduction in the tidal volume will lead inevitably to ventilatory failure.

The fraction of the forced vital capacity expired in 1 second (FEV_1) expressed as a percentage of the FVC is a useful index of the airways resistance (Fig. 4.2). A normal subject should be able to achieve greater than 75%, while a value less than 50% denotes severe airways narrowing which may be associated with ventilatory failure in the postoperative period because of an unacceptably high workload of breathing.

In addition to the foregoing assessments, it may be of value to obtain bacteriological culture of a specimen of sputum together with an indication of the sensitivity of pathogens to antibiotics. Although it is established that there is little merit in the routine use of prophylactic antibiotic therapy in the patient who is undergoing surgery, there may be considerable advantage in delaying operation

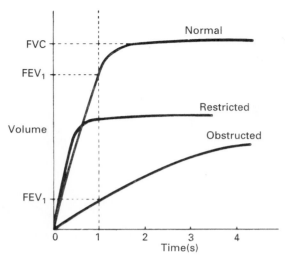

Fig. 4.2   Typical Vitalograph spirograms for the three conditions: (1) normal; (2) restricted: patient with fibrosed lung or limited chest movement as a result of obesity, rib cage disease, pain of an abdominal wound or loss of lung tissue (following pneumonectomy for example); (3) obstructed: patient with airways narrowing such as asthma. Note that only in the obstructed condition is there a delay in the ability to expel gas from the lungs rapidly. Thus, FEV_1 as a proportion of FVC is a useful index of airways narrowing.

for 5–7 days to allow the physiotherapist to institute breathing exercises to promote the expectoration of sputum, and to enable antibiotic therapy to reduce the amount of bacterial contamination.

HEART DISEASE

Most patients with heart disease withstand the pharmacological and physiological stresses of general anaesthesia successfully. Nevertheless, the diseased heart is at risk during anaesthesia and in the postoperative period for a number of important reasons.

Arrhythmia. The patient with an ischaemic myocardium may exhibit abnormal patterns of electrical conduction in the heart muscle which may be aggravated during anaesthesia, either because of a direct effect of the drugs used or as a consequence of inadvertent hypoxia.

Myocardial failure. The failing heart has a reduced ability to compensate for abnormal stresses or hypoxia during or after surgery, adjustments to blood loss and transfusion, and the circulatory disturbances associated with the institution of intermittent positive pressure ventilation.

Previous infarction. Anaesthesia and operation may highlight ischaemia and enhance the risk of another infarct, surgery occurring during the acute stages of recovery from myocardial infarction (the first 3 weeks) being associated with mortality in excess of 50%. A recent myocardial infarction is an indication for postponement of surgery which is not urgent, ideally for a period of not less than 12 months.

Important points in preoperative assessment

History. The patterns of previous illness should be noted, with special reference to the frequency of attacks of cardiac failure, the occurrence of, and precipitating factors in, chest pain, the need for admission to hospital and drug therapy. The capacity for exercise should be noted; a patient who gives a history of previous myocardial infarction but who has been free of symptoms for the past year presents less risk than the patient who suffers recurring attacks of angina at rest, and for which drug treatment is required, even if there has been no acute episode of infarction.

A history suggestive of myocardial failure such as swelling of the abdomen or ankles or attacks of dyspnoea should be noted. In the patient with stenosis of the mitral valve, a recent history of haemoptysis suggests that the cardiac function may be difficult to control.

The routine clinical examination is important in confirming the impressions obtained from the history. X-ray of the chest will provide information about the size of the heart and its outline appearance, and may also indicate the presence of established pulmonary oedema.

The electrocardiogram should be obtained in all such patients; indeed there is a strong case for undertaking investigation in all patients who are more than 40 years of age irrespective of the presence of symptoms and signs. The ECG should be examined for abnormal rhythm, evidence of ventricular enlargement, ischaemia and infarction if present. It should be remembered that patients who are in fact suffering from myocardial infarction may present in the surgical departments of the hospital with symptoms and signs which misleadingly suggest a surgical emergency, notably peritonitis.

The concentration of electrolytes in the serum of patients with heart disease should be measured before operation. In particular, it should be remembered that treatment with diuretics may cause abnormal losses of potassium; the blood urea concentration may be an important clue to renal impairment in patients with established cardiac failure.

If there is associated or co-existing pulmonary disease it is important to measure the arterial oxygen tension (P_aO_2), and the haemoglobin concentration should be known also.

The presence of mild, uncomplicated, arterial hypertension is not regarded as a contraindication to anaesthesia. In many patients it may be a sign of preoperative anxiety, and a second preoperative assessment or 4-hourly observation over 12 hours may reveal a value within the normal limits. If in doubt, selected cases may be treated by rest in bed and mild sedation for a few days.

More severe hypertension. It is widely accepted that such patients benefit from antihypertensive therapy adjusted as necessary for the period of operation. Where possible, operation may be postponed until the patient has been established on a suitable antihypertensive regimen.

Cardiac decompensation will necessitate active treatment with digitalis, diuretics and other appropriate measures.

DIABETES

Diabetes mellitus remains very common and is a demanding challenge in the surgical patient. In addition to the need to control the blood sugar and acid–base balance, patients have an increased risk of vascular and renal disease, neuropathy and retinopathy and an increased risk of infection, including infection of surgical wounds.

As a rule patients who are controlled by diet alone present little difficulty. Those who receive oral hypoglycaemic drugs should continue to take these although some hypoglycaemics (for example, chlorpropamide) have a prolonged duration of action and may induce hypoglycaemia in the fasting patient. If possible that particular drug should be stopped for at least 24 hours before operation. Blood sugar should be monitored and a 5% glucose infusion given. Only very rarely is it necessary to give insulin and that should only be done on the instructions of an experienced diabetologist. Where insulin is used for the control of diabetes the patient is usually treated from one of a variety of published guidelines. A common practice is to commence an infusion of 500 ml of 10% glucose to which has been added 1 g of potassium chloride and 10 units of insulin, all given over 6 hours. This programme can be repeated until the patient is able to return to a normal dietary intake with the restoration of the previous insulin regimen. This plan is based on a scheme introduced by Professor Alberti. The blood glucose concentration should be monitored at least every 3 hours during operation and into the postoperative period. The balance of action should be directed towards maintaining the patient in a relatively hyperglycaemic state rather than risk hypoglycaemia. Poorly controlled diabetics require expert care and surgery should be postponed, unless there is an emergency, for careful management with the help of a diabetologist. Sometimes the elimination of infection can enable a greater control of the diabetic state.

OTHER DISEASES

The preparation and management of patients undergoing procedures for the treatment of endocrine disorders such as phaeochromocytoma, Conn's syndrome, etc. are outside the scope of this book. Patients who have received or are receiving corticosteroids may suffer from suppression of adrenal function necessitating the administration of hydrocortisone 100 mg i.v. or i.m. at least twice daily for 48 hours or until reasonably conventional oral intake can be resumed. If there is any suggestion of adrenocortical insufficiency (typically hypotension that is otherwise unexplained) additional hydrocortisone should be given i.v. even if a regimen of hydrocortisone has already been commenced.

Patients receiving sedative or tranquillizing drugs

These can affect the course of anaesthesia in one of two ways. Patients receiving benzodiazepines or phenothiazines may have reduced requirements for thiopentone and other intravenous induction agents. Thus arterial hypotension and prolonged recovery may follow the administration of the usual dose of an intravenous induction agent if the patient's drug history is not known. On the other hand patients who are habituated to alcohol or to barbiturates may be resistant to normal doses of anaesthetic agents and induction may prove more difficult; this is the result of enzyme induction in the liver with excessively rapid breakdown of the anaesthetic drug.

The monoamine oxidase inhibitor group of drugs used in the treatment of depression may cause severe hypertension, particularly after amphetamine-like drugs. Abnormal reactions to narcotics such as hypotension, hypertension and hyperpyrexia may occur also. Such drugs may be associated with delayed recovery of consciousness after general anaesthesia and with liver damage.

When the patient is examined fully, the overall picture of his physical status may be established. The American Society of Anaesthesiologists classifies physical status in the preoperative period as follows:

Class 1: a normal healthy patient
Class 2: a patient with a mild systemic disease
Class 3: a patient with a severe systemic disease which limits activity but which is not incapacitating.
Class 4: a patient with an incapacitating disease that is a constant threat to life
Class 5: a moribund patient not expected to survive 24 hours with or without operation.

This method of grading the patient is often helpful in impressing on all concerned the necessity for energetic preoperative treatment or, occasionally, for postponing operative treatment.

The purpose of the operation and an outline of the method of anaesthesia should be explained to the patient or his parent and *written permission for anaesthesia must always be obtained.* In the UK, an individual of 16 years of age or more may give consent for treatment without the authority of a parent or guardian provided that he is capable of understanding what the treatment involves. The consent of a parent or guardian should be obtained, however, when the patient is under 16 years of age. In an emergency every reasonable effort should be made to obtain written consent, but if the patient is unconscious, for example, or relatives are not readily available, essential treatment should not be withheld. The consent form should be kept in the patient's record folder and should be checked by the anaesthetist.

ROUTINE PREPARATION

It is essential to ensure that every patient goes to theatre with an empty stomach. There is a small but significant number of deaths each year as a result of vomiting or regurgitation during or immediately after anaesthesia. All these deaths must be regarded as preventable. Normally, no food or fluid is given to the patient by mouth for a period of at least 4 hours before operation. In addition, it is essential to ensure that the patient knows why this is being done and that he does not eat or drink from stores in his locker.

It may not be possible to observe the period of fasting when an emergency operation has to be undertaken shortly after a meal has been ingested. Also, a 4-hour period of fasting may not constitute a guarantee that the stomach is empty in conditions where the stomach fills up from below, for example in intestinal obstruction, or when emptying of the stomach is delayed, notably following injury. In the past, many remedies have been advocated to deal with the problem of the full stomach or the more sinister sequelae. These include forced emesis, aspiration through a wide-bore tube and the insertion of blockers to occlude the outlet from the stomach. None of these measures can be recommended, however, although it is of importance to consider the use of antacid therapy to neutralize gastric acidity. Magnesium trisilicate BPC 15 ml or sodium citrate (0.3 M) 20 ml can be given before operation in an attempt to minimize the acidity of gastric contents, thus reducing the risk of aspiration pneumonitis. In the injured patient, metoclopramide (Maxolon) 10–20 mg i.v. may facilitate gastric emptying to the small bowel.

The bladder and bowel should be emptied. Where major bowel surgery is contemplated, enemata may have been given and some patients, particularly those undergoing gynaecological or urological surgery, will have a urethral catheter in place before operation or shortly after anaesthesia has been induced.

Artificial teeth, contact lenses, rings, hairpins and other objects liable to harm the patient should be removed.

5. Intravenous therapy

The ability to set up an intravenous infusion quickly and confidently is a useful skill for any doctor and an essential one for the anaesthetist, who may have to do so under very difficult conditions.

In many countries there is a variety of needle-in-cannula designs. Factors influencing choice include ease of availability and cost; it is generally advisable to use the same type of equipment regularly, because familiarity with the design improves the chances of success in venepuncture and facilitates connection to the appropriate giving set without inadvertent leakage of the patient's blood.

When a vein is cannulated in a conscious patient it is considerate to infiltrate a small quantity of local anaesthetic solution (1% lignocaine) subcutaneously to anaesthetize the site for skin puncture. A topical eutectic mixture of local anaesthetics may be useful as an alternative.

Usually, the anaesthetist requires an infusion which will allow a rapid controllable flow for a relatively short period — perhaps 24 hours. For this purpose short plastic cannulae are ideal. When an infusion is expected to run for several days, a longer polythene cannula is more suitable. Long, narrow-bore tubing offers considerable resistance to the flow of fluid into the vein and the infusion takes place at a slower rate. When electrolytes are being replaced or when more irritant solutions are delivered into larger, free running veins, these considerations are not important. Nutrient infusions, however, being more viscous, should be administered through a wide cannula.

The site chosen for the venepuncture is of considerable importance (Fig. 5.1). The veins of the antecubital fossa, although very tempting and usually of considerable size, are less suitable for infusion during an operation. Movement of the elbow tends to displace the tip or impede the flow through the cannula and other sites are

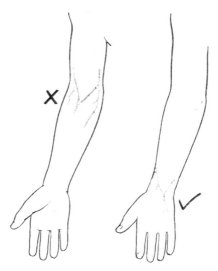

Fig. 5.1   Possible sites for setting up infusions. If the veins round the wrist and the back of the hand are chosen, greater mobility of the limb is possible without dislodging the needle or cannula.

preferred. Among these are the veins at the wrist and on the back of the hand. An infusion inserted here is readily accessible during the operation and injections can be made to it without disturbing the surgical procedure. The wrist can be splinted easily, if necessary, although often this is undesirable, and after operation the patient may be allowed full movement of the hand, provided that care is taken to secure the cannula at the point at which it enters the skin. Normally, in a right-handed person, it is preferable to set up an infusion in the left hand. This point is often overlooked.

As a rule, the leg should not be used for infusions as this may cause phlebitis, particularly if irritant solutions are used or if the infusion has been in existence for more than 48 hours. As the venous blood flow in the leg is less rapid than in the arms, and the leg veins are of larger size, leg vein thrombosis is more likely to occur and may be followed by serious consequences such as pulmonary embolism.

Before setting up an intravenous infusion the doctor should ensure that everything, from the container of infusion fluid to the swabs and tape to secure the cannula, is immediately to hand. It is wise to secure a loop of the giving set at the site of connection to the cannula to prevent traction on the cannula (Fig. 5.2).

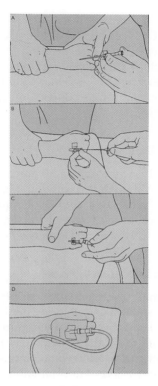

Fig. 5.2   Peripheral intravenous cannulation.

THE CHOICE OF INFUSION FLUID

For short-term management during anaesthesia and for the first 2 days of the postoperative period, it is important to remember that the patient who is deprived of oral intake has an average daily need of about 2.5 litres of water, 140 mmol of sodium and 100 mmol of chloride. Assuming that the patient is in a satisfactory state of fluid and electrolyte balance before operation, other ion losses, such as in the case of potassium and calcium, can be ignored. Water losses may be increased substantially in a warm environment or where there are prolonged losses from the lungs as a result of the inhalation of dry gas during anaesthesia, or from serous surfaces during long operative procedures.

These simple guidelines would not be adequate for the management of the patient who is incapable of a normal oral intake for periods extending beyond 48 hours or for those who may suffer abnormal losses of water and electrolytes, for example from fistulae. For such patients, and indeed for all patients who are undergoing parenteral fluid therapy, a carefully maintained fluid and electrolyte balance chart is the basis of good management.

The choice of infusion fluid depends on the indications for the infusion.

Glucose and distilled water

Glucose injection 5% w/v contains 50 grams of anhydrous glucose per litre of water. Although the solution contains 190 calories per litre, it is of little value as a source of nutrition in the surgical patient, and is used as a means of infusing the requirement of water, without electrolyte, as an isotonic solution.

Sodium chloride injection 0.9% w/v

This solution, sometimes referred to as 'normal saline', contains 150 mmol of both sodium and chloride per litre.

It will be appreciated that the daily requirements of water, sodium and chloride are more than adequately met by the traditional postoperative regimen for an average adult of 1.5–2 litres of 5% dextrose in water and 1 litre of normal saline, although the chloride content is greater than necessary.

Compound sodium lactate injection (Hartmann's solution: Ringer lactate solution)

This solution, sometimes called 'balanced salt solution', contains 131 mmol of sodium, 5 mmol of potassium, 2 mmol of calcium, 111 mmol of chloride and 29 mmol of bicarbonate (as lactate) per litre. The solution is designed to be almost identical in composition to the patient's extracellular fluid. It follows, therefore, that this would be a more suitable solution to use for routine maintenance therapy than normal saline, but the almost universal preference for the latter is traditional and, in practice, there is no serious objection to this. Hartmann's solution is preferred by most anaesthetists as a 'background infusion' during anaesthesia itself for procedures which are expected to last for longer than 30 minutes. Provided that renal function is normal, the recommended practice is to give 1 litre of Hartmann's solution in the first hour of anaesthesia and 500 ml per hour thereafter, in addition to fluid losses which should be replaced with whole blood, packed cells or another plasma expander as appropriate.

During anaesthesia, several hormonal changes occur which have important implications for fluid and electrolyte balance. There is substantial and inappropriate secretion of antidiuretic hormone (ADH) while the adrenal cortex increases its production of aldosterone. ADH inhibits renal secretion of free water (water unaccompanied by ions in isotonic concentration), whereas aldosterone promotes the retention of sodium. Because of these factors, water as 5% dextrose solution and normal saline should not be given in amounts which exceed the anticipated losses. In the presence of satisfactory renal function, however, Hartmann's solution is capable of maintaining the composition and volume of the extracellular fluid while excesses can still be excreted by the kidney.

In the presence of renal disease, and in patients with myocardial failure, parenteral fluid therapy must be approached with caution. In broad terms it can be said that the administration of fluids should be restricted to the anticipated losses only, and even then careful monitoring of the cardiovascular responses to fluid infusion is essential.

Transfusion under pressure

Under certain circumstances it may be desirable to administer fluids, particularly blood, under pressure. Two methods are shown. A second chamber of the giving set containing a ball valve may be compressed to force the fluid into the patient (Fig. 5.3). This method should be used if the fluid is in a rigid container. Alternatively, a compressible cuff may be placed around an infusion bag.

When it is desired to infuse fluid into a child with fine veins, or to give a drug in carefully metered doses to any patient, a specially designed infusion pump may be employed (Fig. 5.4).

Guidance on blood transfusion

In 1995 the Clinical Resource Audit Group* of the National Health Service in Scotland produced a major consensus document

---

*The Scottish Office. National Health Service in Scotland (1995) Optimal use of donor blood. CRAG Secretariat, St Andrew's House, Edinburgh EH1 3DG.

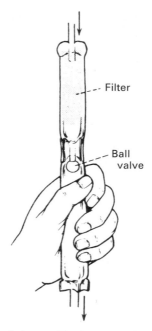

Fig. 5.3   Pressure transfusion set. The lower chamber is allowed to fill with blood and when the full chamber is again compressed the ball occludes the upper outlet and blood is forced down the tubing to the patient.

entitled *Optimal Use of Donor Blood*. This is a useful resource for those who wish to study blood transfusion in greater detail. In particular, it gives an up-to-date list of various published guidelines and consensus statements on transfusion practice.

It is surprisingly difficult to obtain agreement between doctors on the true indications for blood transfusion. For years the criteria were considered to be relatively unimportant provided that supplies from donors were available. In the wake of the AIDS crisis the matter has assumed a new importance.

Often blood is transfused when it has been lost, but many patients who have been in good health before operation can sustain a loss of up to 25% of the circulating blood volume without difficulty provided that some type of appropriate fluid replacement has been given. Blood may be given before operation to correct anaemia. In this case concentrated cells are often used, but whole blood may be infused slowly where concentrated cells are not readily available. Acute haemorrhage may be an indication for whole

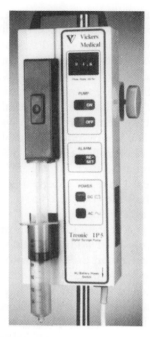

Fig. 5.4   Infusion (syringe) pump.

blood, although increasingly blood banks offer concentrated cells
unless there is a specific request for fresh whole blood. On occasion, a proportion of the measured blood loss may be replaced by
the use of Hartmann's solution or a suitable blood volume
expander such as plasma, dextran, etc. (see pp. 75–76). When an
anaesthetist commences the administration of blood during anaesthesia, he must ensure that the bags or packs of blood being transfused are those which have been previously grouped and
cross-matched for the patient. Careful checking of the name and
group on the bottle with those on the patient's case sheet is essential
to avoid accidents. This is particularly important during anaesthesia
when transfusion reactions are more difficult to recognize.
Unexplained tachycardia, hypotension and oozing at the operation
site may indicate the use of the wrong blood. The late consequences
of a mismatched transfusion are renal failure and jaundice as a result
of haemolysis. It is important also to remember that the potassium
concentration in the serum of the stored blood may be much greater
than that of the patient's serum, and that the pH is low.

Blood stored in a refrigerator will be transfused at a temperature below that of the body, the difference varying with the time lapse between removal and transfusion and the rate of transfusion. With slow transfusions of relatively small amounts of blood, the low temperature of the blood is of little consequence. When large quantities of cold blood are transfused rapidly, however, a severe reduction in body temperature may result, leading to cardiac arrest. Steps must be taken, therefore, to warm the blood to body temperature. This is done by passing the blood through a heated and thermostatically controlled coil (Fig. 5.5).

In the transfusion of blood for the treatment of anaemia, it should be remembered that the elderly and those with a predisposition to cardiac failure may be placed at risk from excessive expansion of the circulating blood volume. Thus, slow infusion with careful monitoring is essential. Citrate-phosphate-dextrose (CPD) is the most frequently used additive to blood and allows it to be stored for 4–5 weeks. Blood preserved with CPD can be stored at temperatures in the range of 2–6°C. Such a preparation has few platelets and is deficient in factors V, VIII and XI. Factors IX and X will be deficient after about 1 week of storage. Older CPD blood becomes deficient in 2, 3 diphosphoglycerate (2, 3 DPG) in the later phase of storage. It should be realized that if 2, 3 DPG is substantially depleted in a blood transfusion, there would be no net improvement in oxygen carriage as a result of treatment.

Blood filters

Although the standard infusion apparatus for blood incorporates a fine mesh which acts as a filter for aggregates which may have formed during the storage period, there is evidence that small aggregates can pass through these filters. These particles may form small emboli, notably in the lungs. This may contribute to or cause the 'shock lung' syndrome. Where blood or red cells have to be given the giving set should incorporate a 170 μm filter.

Risk of infection from blood

Transfused blood can be a source of infection to the patient. Viral B hepatitis and AIDS are the best known examples, but malaria, syphilis, cytomegalovirus and the Epstein–Barr virus may be problems also. With a high quality blood transfusion system the risks are minimal, but it is important to be aware of how the blood has

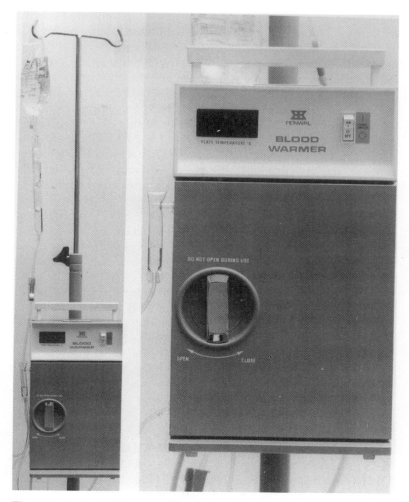

Fig. 5.5 An electrically operated blood warmer ready for use.

been obtained and how the blood and the patient have been screened beforehand.

Plasma

The need for plasma proteins, as opposed to whole blood, arises in two circumstances. Reconstituted dried plasma obtained from small donor pools may be transfused while blood is being obtained and cross-matched. This will restore the circulating volume but will not replace the oxygen-carrying capacity of the blood which has been lost. In patients who are hypovolaemic and in electrolyte imbalance, plasma may be used to expand the circulatory volume and ensure adequate renal perfusion before administering aqueous electrolyte solutions; full plasma is rich in potassium. Even when plasma has been obtained from small groups of donors, there remains the risk of transmitting serum hepatitis. The manifestations of this may vary from a minor upset in liver function to severe jaundice and may prejudice the life of a seriously ill patient. For this reason, among others, plasma substitutes have been developed. It is possible to give solutions of albumin, salt-poor albumin or, most commonly, a solution known as the plasma protein fraction (PPF). PPF is obtained by a pasteurization process which results in the removal by precipitation of the globulin fraction and viruses. Thus the hazard of serum hepatitis is greatly reduced if a solution of this type is used.

Fresh frozen plasma is rich in clotting factors and its use is reserved for circumstances — most commonly in association with massive blood transfusion — in which the clotting mechanism is likely to be impaired. Cryoprecipitate, which is used principally in the treatment of haemophilia, is also very rich in clotting factors. Concentrated platelet preparations are given in the treatment of platelet deficiency.

Plasma substitutes

A plasma substitute such as dextran (Dextran, Dextraven, Macrodex) may be given if blood or plasma is not readily available. This is a sugar solution containing large molecules (average molecular weight 70 000) with a high osmotic pressure which acts as a plasma expander. A reduction in postoperative phlebothrombosis is also claimed where Dextran 70 has been given during and after operation. Rheomacrodex is a solution of lesser molecular weight (average = 40 000). Although it has a short half-life of about 3 hours in the body, it will restore the blood volume and may increase renal output by reducing the viscosity of blood after a considerable amount of blood has been given. However, excessive quantities result in the production of a highly viscid urine, tubular obstruction and a form of postrenal failure. A gelatine in saline (Gelofusine, Haemaccel) solution remains with the circulation for

6–12 hours. There are few complications associated with the use of such solutions.

Fluorocarbons and hydroxyethyl starch are other substances which have potential for plasma volume expansion.

BLOOD LOSS ESTIMATIONS

Often it is not clear when to begin blood replacement and when to discontinue it. Ideally, of course, blood volume should be measured and haematocrit readings may be useful also. Often, however, such measurements are impracticable and the value of haemoglobin or haematocrit measurements will depend to a large extent on the degree of haemoconcentration or haemodilution.

By weighing the swabs which have been used during operation and comparing them with dry swabs, it is possible to calculate the amount of blood which has been lost. It is also possible to wash the blood from the swabs and, by using a colorimeter, to measure the quantity lost.

When blood is lost the peripheral circulation is reduced and the blood flow through the extremities, as detected by the plethysmograph (pp. 235–237), decreases. Only when this process can no longer compensate for the haemorrhage does the heart rate increase. When the increase is no longer adequate to compensate for the blood loss, the arterial pressure decreases. This is shown in Figure 5.6.

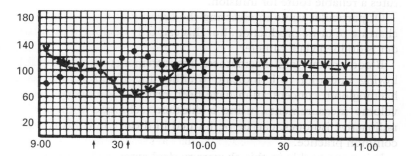

Fig. 5.6   Arterial systolic pressure (mm Hg: V) and pulse rate (beat min^{-1}: ●) measured in an anaesthetized patient who lost through haemorrhage approximately 1100 ml of blood (arrows). Replacement transfusion was commenced at 0930 h and 1000 ml had been given by 0945 h. In this instance pressure and rate were restored very nearly to the values noted before haemorrhage. With greater losses (and replacement) some degree of persisting hypotension and tachycardia might be encountered.

When blood loss is overt and appears likely to continue, it is desirable that replacement should be commenced before the onset of tachycardia and certainly before the arterial pressure has decreased markedly. Similarly, provided that other causes of tachycardia and hypotension can be excluded, it is desirable to continue the transfusion until the arterial pressure and the pulse rate have returned to normal. Some indication of the adequacy of blood replacement can be gained by observing the filling of the neck veins when the patient is lying flat or with the head slightly raised. The central venous pressure (CVP), if measured, may be a useful additional guide. Provided that myocardial function is adequate, the usual response to haemorrhage is a reduction in CVP. If the heart is failing, however, the effects of haemorrhage could cause an increase in CVP. As a general rule the anaesthetist will use knowledge of the patient's preoperative state to interpret the changes; sudden myocardial failure would not be expected during haemorrhage if the patient was young or middle-aged and was known to have good myocardial function before operation.

An additional problem in interpreting CVP measurements during anaesthesia is that change of position of the patient, intra-abdominal pressure from packs, and retractors may cause artifacts. For this reason the value of CVP measurement is seen by some anaesthetists as being not worth the time, effort and invasion involved. If, however, the patient is likely to benefit from monitoring of CVP in the postoperative period, the venous catheter should be inserted during anaesthesia; in addition to its value for monitoring it constitutes a reliable route for infusion.

Of particular value in assessing the severity of blood loss is the charting of urine production, but this can only be done if the bladder is drained via a catheter.

Blood volume and haematocrit measurements on the day following operation will indicate whether the blood volume and haemoglobin concentration have been restored to normal. Blood volume measurements, using a dilution technique with dye or radioactive isotopes, can be performed in theatre but this is not a common practice.

It is not possible in this chapter to deal extensively with all the problems associated with intravenous therapy. Remember when setting up an infusion to consider what you are trying to replace and the most logical method of replacing it. Never give blood if it is not indicated but do not hesitate to use blood where it is indicated, bearing in mind the replacement of blood volume and haemoglobin with its oxygen-carrying capacity. Where possible, measure the blood loss. Knowledge of the electrolyte values in the blood will allow the correct amount and type of electrolyte to be replaced. In the same way, acid-base measurements allow acidosis or alkalosis to be corrected.

In transfusing small children, note that their blood volume is approximately 110 ml/kg body weight and that 500 ml of blood to a small child may represent a considerable proportion of the normal blood volume. Try neither to under-transfuse nor to over-transfuse. On the one hand the heart has to beat faster to compensate for the deficiency in blood volume; on the other hand the administration of excessive quantities of blood will impose a strain on the heart.

The control of intravenous infusions in general is a matter requiring cooperation between surgeon, anaesthetist and laboratory. Remember that if the need for large quantities of blood is anticipated, the blood bank must be warned in plenty of time as there may be difficulty in providing the requirements at a moment's notice.

'Massive' blood transfusion

The transfusion of large quantities of blood can cause a series of problems which may tax the clinical judgement of the anaesthetist and the laboratory services of the hospital. It is difficult to give an agreed definition of massive transfusion but it may be taken as the administration of somewhere between 4 and 10 units of blood. The risks are:

- *Hypothermia.* This may be lessened by the appropriate warming of blood and by the use of space blankets to prevent the patient's body temperature from decreasing too rapidly.
- *Acidosis.* This may be a combined effect of tissue acidosis or a result of hypoxia associated with the condition requiring transfusion in the first instance. In addition, acidosis is a feature of citrate intoxication, a problem to be remembered when citrate has been used as part of the preservative. Where large transfusions are anticipated, some hospitals prefer to use heparinized blood which avoids the problem of citrate intoxication.
- *Hyperkalaemia.* Stored blood is a potent source of potassium ion. In association with hyperkalaemia there may be a reduction in the serum magnesium concentration.

- *Loss of clotting factors.* Patients who have had massive transfusions are likely to be deficient in factors V, VII and X and in circulating platelets. The solution to this is to administer fresh frozen plasma or concentrated platelets, or both.

6. The administration of a general anaesthetic

An anaesthetic can be divided into two phases: *induction* and *maintenance*. These may merge imperceptibly or there may be a fairly obvious demarcation between them. Induction of anaesthesia is considered to last from the moment when the anaesthetic is commenced until the requisite level of anaesthesia has been achieved for whatever operation is contemplated. This may take a few minutes or a considerable time, depending upon the method chosen and the skill of the anaesthetist.

INDUCTION OF ANAESTHESIA

This is usually achieved by intravenous injection of suitable agents or by inhalation of nitrous oxide, or vapours of volatile anaesthetic liquids. Before selecting a method, several questions must be answered:

- What is the safest method of induction?
- What is most pleasant for the patient?
- Which is the easiest and most practicable method under the circumstances?

The safety of each method lies in the avoidance of the complications associated with induction. These are: regurgitation as the oesophageal sphincter relaxes; hypoxaemia (associated with coughing, bucking or laryngeal spasm); respiratory depression; and a decrease in arterial pressure resulting in circulatory insufficiency. For example, the inhalation of diethyl ether avoids the risk of sudden respiratory or cardiovascular depression, although the relative risk of coughing, etc. is greater. A rapid induction with intravenous thiopentone followed by suxamethonium may hasten the conditions for tracheal intubation, thus minimizing the risks of regurgitation, although respiratory and cardiovascular depression are

81

more likely. Paradoxically, the rapid induction techniques are still associated with a short period of risk of regurgitation at a time when the protective reflexes have been totally abolished. Thus there is no easy rule-of-thumb in the selection of the technique, and the experience of the anaesthetist and the general condition of the patient are important determinants of the choice.

Intravenous induction of anaesthesia

The drugs normally used are described in Chapter 2. Here we describe induction with thiopentone.

This drug should be made up in a 2.5% solution in water. A suitable vein with an indwelling cannula, on the dorsum of the hand preferably, provides the route of injection and 1–2 ml of solution is injected. Thereafter, the injection is halted and a few moments are allowed for the drug to circulate. The patient is then asked whether there is pain in the limb, at or below the point of injection. This is an essential precaution. If this test has been negative and the patient has not complained of pain, a further 2–3 ml should be injected, after which there should be a pause, and a further 2–3 ml of solution injected.

It is essential not to have fixed ideas as to the dose of thiopentone to be given before starting the injection. Small quantities should be injected at suitable intervals until the patient loses consciousness. If the patient is ill and has a slow circulation, longer pauses will be required between each 2–3 ml injection to allow the drug to circulate. The total dose of drug required to produce unconsciousness may vary widely, the ill, debilitated patient requiring perhaps 100 mg, the wrestler with a taste for alcohol requiring little less than 1 g. It is a popular practice to ask the patient to count, and when counting ceases sleep is assumed. However, some patients may continue counting in an automatic fashion beyond the point at which they can respond sensibly to questions asked in conversation. Many anaesthetists, therefore, prefer to speak to the patient and to note the point at which there is no answer.

When sleep has ensued, it is normally advisable to cease the injection of thiopentone, as the drug is intended only to induce sleep and further administration may depress the myocardium. The induction is continued by administration of 70% nitrous oxide in oxygen and, if necessary, a volatile agent such as halothane may be added. If halothane is chosen, increments of 0.5% are added to reach perhaps 3–4% depending on the response of the patient (see description of *overpressure*, p. 4), but this concentration will be maintained only for a short time. In the case of enflurane, which is less potent, a higher concentration will be required. Sometimes a limitation in the case of this drug is the maximum output of the commonly used 'Enflurotec' vaporizer at 5% (v/v).

Inhalation induction of anaesthesia

The patient is asked to breathe a mixture of 70% nitrous oxide in oxygen. This is continued until consciousness is lost as evidenced by loss of the eyelash reflex or the onset of a breathing pattern which is regular in rate or depth. A volatile agent, usually halothane, is now added in gradually increasing percentage, as described above, until the required level of anaesthesia is reached. Inhalation induction is more difficult with enflurane or isoflurane but relatively easy with sevoflurane.

Pre-oxygenation

This practice both precedes and accompanies intravenous induction of anaesthesia. If 100% oxygen is breathed for 2–3 minutes, a large part of the nitrogen in the lungs will be washed out and replaced by oxygen. With this reserve in hand the safe period of apnoea may be prolonged about four-fold in comparison with the patient who has breathed air only, and tracheal intubation may be accomplished without hypoxia.

It is wise to practise the technique of pre-oxygenation; although it is possibly unnecessary for many patients, it is always a valuable safeguard.

As we have now induced anaesthesia to a light level, administration of inhalation agents will continue until the anaesthesia is considered to be deep enough for the operation to be commenced. Obviously the criteria will vary with the particular operation and the degree of muscular relaxation required for its performance. No mention has been made here of the use of muscle relaxants, and these will be considered separately as they involve the problems of assisted or controlled ventilation.

Before we can decide rationally when to reduce the concentration of volatile anaesthetics and judge that the patient is at a level of anaesthesia adequate for any particular operation, we must consider the signs of anaesthesia, as they give a guide to the level of unconsciousness which has been or must be attained.

THIS SIGNS OF ANAESTHESIA

The stages and planes of anaesthesia, as described and taught normally, are those formulated by Guedel. They applied to ether anaesthesia after premedication with atropine but are still a valuable guide for other types of anaesthesia and should be committed to memory. A modified table of Guedel's signs is shown in Figure 6.1.

Many students are rather puzzled to see that the classic stages and signs about which they have read are not in evidence when modern anaesthetic techniques are used. There are, however, good reasons for this. We have discussed earlier (p. 7) the division of anaesthesia into its three parts: sleep, analgesia and muscular relaxation. It is this division of anaesthesia into its component parts and the use of specific drugs to produce them which has revolutionized anaesthesia compared with Guedel's time. One may, for instance, produce apnoea, which does not occur until stage IV

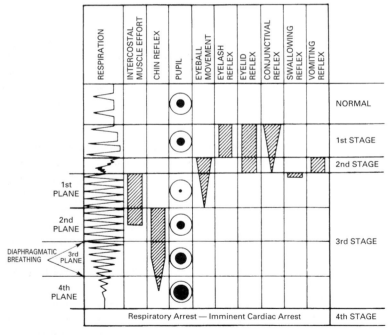

Fig. 6.1   Stages and planes of anaesthesia (after Guedel 1937). Many of these signs may be used to estimate the depth of unconsciousness resulting from other causes, e.g. head injuries.

in Guedel's classification, by the use of myoneural blockade without having produced either unconsciousness or indeed any analgesia. Similarly, it is possible, by rapid injection of a barbiturate, to produce apnoea, although the patient will respond to a painful stimulus. It is for this reason that, using modern anaesthetic techniques, the anaesthetist must depend on additional signs to identify the depth of anaesthesia.

Loss of consciousness

When thiopentone or propofol are used it is not difficult to demonstrate that the patient has lost consciousness; for example he may be asked to count. Using inhalation methods, the distinction is not quite so clear but the return of automatic (regular) breathing is a sure sign that consciousness has been lost. In addition, the loss of the eyelid reflex — the eyelash is stroked with the finger and the eyelid no longer closes — is a valuable guide to loss of consciousness. A further, but seldom used, test is to ask the patient to hold one arm in the air and when the arm falls to his side he is asleep.

When anaesthesia is continued with nitrous oxide and a volatile supplement in oxygen, the problem of inadvertent regaining of consciousness seldom arises. On rare occasions, patients in whom anaesthesia is maintained with nitrous oxide, oxygen and a muscle relaxant may complain that they remember incidents during an operation. This has occurred when no sedative premedication has been used, when a limited dose of thiopentone has been given for induction, and when anaesthesia has been maintained using nitrous oxide and more than 33% of oxygen. In obstetric anaesthesia, the risk of depressing the baby has resulted in a tendency to reduce the dosage of narcotics and volatile anaesthetics, and it is in this context that the problem of awareness occurs most frequently.

The use of hyoscine in premedication in place of atropine is believed by some to reduce this incidence of awareness during anaesthesia.

The routine use of a supplementary volatile agent with nitrous oxide and oxygen should abolish awareness in surgical practice but is associated with a slower recovery of consciousness.

The return of the eyelash reflex and movements of the eyelids and eyebrows in a patient who has received a myoneural blocking drug (see below) should suggest that the patient requires supplementation of the anaesthetic.

Assessment of analgesia (sensory blockade)

Here we are looking for the normal physiological reactions of the conscious person to pain, modified according to the degree of analgesia present and whether or not a muscle relaxant has been used.

Withdrawal from the painful stimulus. This may take the form of gross movement — a hand may be withdrawn from the surgeon's knife or the patient may draw up his knee. Such movement results when the level of anaesthesia is too light and a severe stimulus is applied. When the depth of anaesthesia is just insufficient for the operation to be performed and when a muscle relaxant has been used, the reaction may be restricted to slight movement of the fingers and hand or wrinkling of the forehead. The patient may move his head from side to side in a characteristic rocking fashion.

Phonation. Patients will normally cry out when hurt and, if it is possible during light anaesthesia, some attempt at phonation is usually made. Obviously this is not possible when an endotracheal tube is in place.

Irregular breathing or breath-holding may be signs of inadequate analgesia for the operation being performed. Laryngeal stridor may be included under this heading.

A further group of signs is associated with *sympathetic overactivity* — part of the 'fight or flight' reaction; the skin is seen to be pale, cold and sweating, and heart rate and arterial pressure are increased.

Another important sign is *lachrymation.*

These signs may be found at the beginning of the operation when the surgeon's skin incision is made, during operation if the anaesthetic becomes too light, or in operations where intensely painful stimuli are inflicted at intervals. They are an indication to increase the depth of anaesthesia by increasing the concentration of the volatile agent. If only nitrous oxide and oxygen are administered in the gas mixture, the signs are an indication for the addition of a volatile agent to the mixture or for the administration of small doses of a narcotic.

Within the last two decades there has been a trend towards the use of narcotic drugs injected intravenously to supplement nitrous oxide anaesthesia in patients receiving neuromuscular blocking drugs with artificial ventilation of the lungs. It should be remembered that the MAC of nitrous oxide cannot be achieved under normal atmospheric conditions. Morphine and fentanyl are the most popular drugs for this type of supplementation.

There are three main reasons for giving intravenous narcotics in this way: avoidance of atmospheric pollution, possible greater stability of the cardiovascular system if drugs such as halothane or isoflurane are not given, and the belief (for which there is some experimental evidence in the case of fentanyl) that narcotics may lessen some aspects of the metabolic response to anaesthesia and surgery (see also p. 31).

The disadvantage of using narcotics for maintenance of anaesthesia is the fact that it requires great skill to ensure a steady pharmacological effect throughout the anaesthetic. The MAC concept for inhalation agents offers a convenient guide to likely dose, but there is nothing comparable to the effect of drugs given intravenously. In the wrong hands intravenous maintenance may incur the risk either of awareness because too little anaesthetic has been given or of postoperative respiratory depression from too much.

Is muscular relaxation adequate?

The degree of muscular relaxation needed for any particular operation is a matter which can only be decided by experience and a little foresight.

During diethyl ether anaesthesia, the anaesthetist may look for the signs in Guedel's classification to estimate the degree of muscular relaxation according to the *stage* of anaesthesia. Careful observation of these signs during inhalation anaesthesia will ensure that the appropriate level of anaesthesia is maintained throughout.

When minor procedures, such as the manipulation of a fracture, are to be carried out, it is possible, after anaesthesia has been induced, to test the relaxation in the limb concerned. It must be remembered, however, that, while a limb may be flaccid at rest, when painful manipulation is carried out the muscles may contract.

When myoneural blockade has been produced and ventilation of the lungs is controlled, it may be difficult for the anaesthetist to decide whether relaxation remains adequate. Although breathing may have been abolished by the original dose of muscle relaxant, in many cases the fact that it has not restarted is not of itself a sufficient indication that relaxation remains complete. While ventilation is controlled, the level of carbon dioxide in the blood may be reduced. This, together with central depression by the anaesthetic drugs, may account for continuing apnoea after the effect of the neuromuscular block has lessened. Some guides to the fact that relaxation has lessened are:

- *The surgeon may complain that the patient's muscles are tense.* This is not always a reliable guide as surgeons tend to differ in their estimation of what is adequate relaxation. A particularly courteous surgeon may not wish to cause offence!
- If the anaesthetist observes the surgical wound in the abdomen, he may see that *bowel is being extruded* or that the peritoneum is retracted into the wound, or is tearing as it is being stitched.
- If ventilation is being controlled by manual compression of the reservoir bag, the anaesthetist may notice that the *pressure required to inflate the lungs to the same volume is increasing* and that greater effort has to be used to inflate the lungs with the same volume of gas. If a mechanical ventilator is being used it is possible that, to maintain the same tidal volume, a higher inflation pressure is required; if the ventilator is set to deliver a constant pressure, a reduced volume of gas may be delivered to the patient by the same pressure. These effects are a result of returning tone in the muscles of the chest wall and upper abdomen.
- If the anaesthetist does not appreciate these signs and compensates (for a reduced volume) by increasing the pressure in the reservoir bag, it may be noticed that the *arterial pressure is decreasing* without obvious reason. This is a result of the increased intrathoracic pressure reducing the venous return and, consequently, the cardiac output.
- There may be movement ('chewing') of the tracheal tube or the patient may make *spontaneous respiratory efforts.*

When muscle relaxation is seen to be inadequate on the basis of these signs, the first matter to be considered is whether the level of anaesthesia should be deepened. If a volatile anaesthetic is being given the anaesthetist will have a good guide to this from knowledge of the concentration delivered. If the depth of anaesthesia is thought to be inadequate, a supplementary dose of the muscle relaxant is given intravenously. Increasingly, dosage is controlled by the clinician using a nerve stimulator attached to the patient's forearm. Return of the normal response is taken as an indication for a further supplementary dose of relaxant.

One must consider what signs are most likely to be shown by the patient under the circumstances of any given anaesthetic. If an opiate has been used in premedication and thiopentone has been given early in the procedure, the patient's pupils are likely to be small throughout the anaesthesia in the absence of gross hypoxia or very severe painful stimuli. Similarly, when muscle relaxant drugs have been administered, the eyeball will remain fixed while they are acting.

Provided that the patient is adequately relaxed and hyperventilation is undertaken, some anaesthetists consider that the signs suggestive of inadequate analgesia are not of importance. However, this is precisely the situation in which a later complaint of awareness during surgery may occur. On the other hand it has been shown that even under deep levels of anaesthesia where there are no outward signs that the patient is receiving painful stimuli, such stimuli in fact do reach the cerebral cortex, and there is little indication that the patient is any the worse for this. The only method of blocking the passage of these impulses to the brain is by regional nerve block, that is blocking the impulses as they pass along nerves before they reach the spinal cord.

THE FURTHER MAINTENANCE AND CONCLUSION OF ANAESTHESIA

We have dealt at some length with the recognition of various signs during anaesthesia. If one understands what to look for and recognize during anaesthesia, then appropriate action can be taken. Thus if the patient is inadequately anaesthetized, further increments of the intravenous analgesic or an increased concentration of the volatile agent can be given. If muscle relaxation is inadequate appropriate measures can be taken and, if ventilation is inadequate, this can be augmented. Early recognition of problems and prompt treatment will ensure that anaesthesia continues smoothly.

We may, however, consider in further detail the administration of two types of anaesthetic.

Spontaneous breathing with inhalation agents

Anaesthesia may be induced by either intravenous or inhalation methods as mentioned in the section on induction of anaesthesia. The patient will have been anaesthetized to the level appropriate for the particular operation and the anaesthetist will watch for the signs which indicate that this level has been reached. He will then keep a regular check on the signs of anaesthesia at the level which he has chosen and, provided that they are maintained, a low concentration of vapour such as 0.5–1% halothane will suffice for a prolonged period. Towards the end of operation the level of anaesthesia may be lightened, but the extent of this will depend on the depth to which anaesthesia has been carried and the nature of the operation. Thus if nitrous oxide, oxygen and halothane have been given, halothane may be discontinued as the wound is being closed. However, it is a matter of judgement and experience to ensure that the level of anaesthesia does not lighten excessively before the end of the surgical procedure. While it is desirable to have a patient regain consciousness within a few minutes of the termination of the operation, it is a risky procedure to try to maintain a very light level of anaesthesia, since it is at this level that vomiting, coughing and laryngeal spasm are most likely. Thus adequate anaesthesia should be maintained until one is in a position to deal with these complications during recovery from anaesthesia without interrupting the course of the operation.

Controlled ventilation using muscle relaxants

Anaesthesia will usually be induced by the use of an intravenous agent, and a myoneural blocking drug will be given to paralyse the muscles. Thereafter a tracheal tube will be passed and ventilation controlled by manual or mechanical means. During the operation the signs of inadequate analgesia and inadequate ventilation will be sought and the patient observed carefully to ensure that relaxation is adequate. Supplements of the anaesthetic, analgesic or relaxant drugs will be given according to the indications, and these procedures will be continued throughout the operation. Once the peritoneum is closed, the patient, usually still apnoeic, will have to be prepared for the end of the operation and steps are now taken to restore spontaneous ventilation.

If the muscle relaxant is still considered to be acting, as shown by ease in closing the peritoneum, the appropriate antagonist is given. In the case of the non-depolarizing drugs, neostigmine in a dose of 2.5–5 mg i.v. is given. As this drug produces severe bradycardia, marked salivation and possibly bronchospasm, it is preceded by atropine, normally 1.2 mg administered intravenously. If spontaneous breathing does not follow the administration of these drugs, further steps may be necessary in the light of the possible causes of continued apnoea. If hyperventilation of the lung alveoli has occurred during the operation, this is usually detectable as a lower than normal end tidal CO_2 concentration (normally about 5%). A reduced respiratory frequency with maintained oxygenation will gradually allow CO_2 to accumulate to the normal level. If tracheobronchial or pharyngeal suction is undertaken, the passage of the catheter into the trachea or into the pharynx is often sufficient, as a non-specific stimulus, to cause spontaneous breathing. Where excessive depression by narcotic analgesics is suspected, naloxone up to 0.4 mg may be given intravenously as an antagonist. As a rule, however, such drugs should not be necessary if the decision about the dosage of narcotics during surgery has been appropriate.

When an endotracheal tube is in place, tracheobronchial suction, using a sterile catheter through the tube, is undertaken to remove secretions.

As tracheobronchial suction may deplete the lungs' store of oxygen, it is essential to administer oxygen before and after suction to compensate for this. At this stage secretions should be cleared from the pharynx under direct vision using the laryngoscope. Thereafter, the tube is withdrawn from the trachea. Once the pharynx has been aspirated, the same catheter should not be used again in the trachea in case infection is introduced. At this stage the patient may be transferred to a tilting trolley and placed on his side (Figs 6.2, 6.3). Supplementary oxygen, in the range 28–40%, should be given, particularly in patients with cardiovascular or respiratory disease.

When the patient has recovered to a degree which satisfies the anaesthetist it is appropriate to transfer care to the nursing staff in

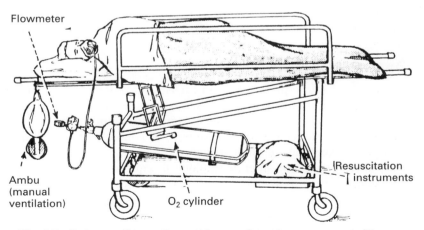

Fig. 6.2   Patient on tilting trolley awaiting transfer to the recovery room. The cylinder of oxygen lies below the trolley and the mechanism for tilting is above the cylinder.

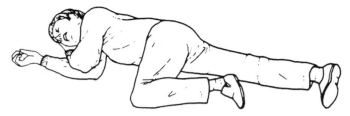

Fig. 6.3   The tonsillar position: the patient lies midway between the lateral and the prone positions, prevented from rolling face downwards by the pillow and the position of the arms and legs.

the recovery room. At all stages in the transfer it is important to remember that responsible supervision of the patient is a continuing obligation.

Before leaving the operating room, if the patient has received muscle relaxant drugs, it is important to check that the patient can put out the tongue or lift the head from the pillow. If this can be done it is likely that the condition is safe for transfer to the recovery room. The increasing use of neuromuscular block monitors has greatly facilitated this aspect of care.

The anaesthetist should never be rushed into starting another anaesthetic before the condition of the previous patient is assured. It is also important to ensure that clear instructions for the patient's immediate recovery room care (oxygen, analgesia, parenteral fluids, care of thoracic drainage, etc.) are transmitted effectively to the recovery room staff.

Awareness and recall

From time to time press attention focuses on reports of patients who complain of having been aware during a general anaesthetic. Quite apart from this representing an apparent failure of the obvious contract between doctor and patient, the consequences of such an event, if genuine, can be harrowing. There may be substantial sleep disturbance and other psychological sequelae such as failure to 'bond' between mother and child if the anaesthetic was given for caesarean section.

It is sometimes claimed that the problem can arise without any clear explanation but the authors doubt this. Sometimes recall may be a consequence of the deliberate use of very light anaesthesia; for example in a desperately shocked patient for a temporary period there is a reluctance to administer any drugs that are likely to reduce further the cardiac output. In most cases, however, recall is a result of technical failure: the disconnection of gas and vapour supplies to breathing systems; the inadvertent exhaustion of a vaporizer supply of volatile anaesthetic; or wrong settings of flow meters and vaporizers.

It is generally believed that recall only occurs in circumstances in which a neuromuscular blocking drug has been given and the patient is unable to achieve spontaneous muscular activity. The 'safeguard' for patients who have not received neuromuscular blocking drugs is that, if the level of anaesthesia is insufficient to suppress awareness, the patient would ultimately be able to leave the operating table, even if no one had noticed any preliminary signs. There is no reason to fear the awful prospect of a paralysed patient who is aware of surrounding events and the pain of a surgical operation. Even under neuromuscular block there are many valid clinical signs of light anaesthesia, never mind awareness. The patient will sweat, the arterial pressure will tend to rise, the pulse rate increase. There is usually the prospect of some breakthrough muscle activity in movement of the eyebrows, chewing on the tracheal tube, an attempted respiratory effort or even the beginnings of the movement of the limbs. At all times the anaesthetist should be moderately confident of having achieved approximately the right level of anaesthesia from a knowledge of MAC and the likelihood that somewhere in the order of 1.3 times MAC is being given, plus a recognition of the effects likely to be produced by drugs that may have been given intravenously such as opioids and benzodiazepines.

There has been something of a burgeoning industry offering various ingenious devices to demonstrate objectively the consequences of an inadequately light anaesthetic. For example, systems have been produced to process the EEG, while others have sought a muscle response through electromyography, and yet another has used the detection of patterns of oesophageal contraction following a physical stimulus to the oesophagus as a monitor. In fact all of these devices can be shown to correlate well with the 'depth' of anaesthesia as signified by the MAC equivalent of the gas and vapour mixture administered, but they are not in themselves able to detect that the patient is capable of recall through awareness. We repeat, however, that the problem of awareness and recall is rare and the circumstances in which it occurs are apparently predictable mishaps.

Where central nervous system depressants have been given, albeit inadequately, it is worth noting that there is a predictable order for the loss of sensation: smell and olfaction are lost at the lightest level of anaesthesia, followed by visual disturbance and some loss of sensation at deeper anaesthesia, and finally the loss of hearing. It is perhaps not surprising, therefore, that if the level of anaesthesia is truly inadequate the patient is more likely to recall speech, music or noise than any other sensation.

7. Endotracheal intubation and endoscopy; the laryngeal mask airway

The technique of laryngoscopy and intubation of the trachea is essential to the practice of anaesthesia. However, these simple skills are of value outside the operating theatre in a variety of circumstances, ranging from resuscitation of the newborn to the first aid management of the patient who has suffered cardiac arrest.

Indications for endotracheal intubation

Maintenance of a clear airway under difficult circumstances

If the anaesthetized patient is to lie on his side, on his face or in the head-down position, it may not be possible to maintain a clear airway using an oropharyngeal airway only. In obese subjects, particularly those who are edentulous, it may even be difficult to maintain the airway during anaesthesia in the supine position. In all these circumstances the insertion of a tracheal tube assures the airway.

Operations on the head, neck, mouth, throat and nose

In most of these procedures the anaesthetist and the surgeon may be competing for access and the use of a face mask is impracticable; a tracheal tube and its connection is much less obtrusive.

Protection of the trachea

The presence of a cuffed tracheal tube prevents materials such as blood, mucus, pus or vomitus from gaining access to the trachea and the lungs. This is of particular importance for operations on the nose and mouth and in patients liable to vomit or regurgitate during anaesthesia, notably in obstetric practice and in patients with intestinal obstruction.

95

Reduction of respiratory dead space

The presence of a tracheal tube will reduce the physiological dead space by 30–40%. This is of particular importance in the small child in whom the use of a face mask might add to the respiratory dead space to such an extent as to cause ventilatory failure.

Facilitation of tracheobronchial toilet

A tracheal tube facilitates the passage of a suction catheter to the trachea and main bronchi for the aspiration of mucus and other undesired material. In the case of a discrete plug of mucus or more solid matter, bronchoscopy may be necessary. This procedure is described later in this chapter. A fibreoptic probe may be inserted via a tracheal tube for inspection of the bronchial tree and suction under direct vision. Once the tracheal tube is in position, fibreoptic endoscopy causes virtually no additional disturbance to the patient.

Controlled ventilation

In most circumstances in which it is intended to undertake artificial ventilation of the lungs by intermittent positive pressure, the presence of a tracheal tube (except in patients in whom tracheostomy has been performed) is essential. However, these comments do not apply to the use of positive pressure ventilation for a few minutes in the resuscitation of the apnoeic patient. In these patients the application of gas under pressure from a face mask (using an Ambu bag for example) is a first essential in treatment, and satisfactory oxygenation of the arterial blood should be restored before tracheal intubation is attempted.

Therapeutic indications for endotracheal intubation

In the care of the unconscious, the absence of an adequate cough reflex warrants tracheal intubation to ensure protection of the airway from liquid material in the pharynx. In addition, the presence of the tube allows tracheobronchial toilet to be carried out at any time. Thus there are indications for endotracheal intubation in patients who have been severely poisoned by respiratory depressants and in patients with head injury and cerebrovascular accidents.

In patients with postoperative respiratory insufficiency, the use of a tracheal tube may reduce the respiratory dead space sufficiently to allow adequate ventilation until recovery of function (by the control of pain or the antagonism of myoneural blockade) has occurred.

In resuscitation of the newborn, the passage of a tracheal tube facilitates artificial ventilation and endotracheal suction. In other forms of resuscitation such as the treatment, after the first few minutes, of cardiac arrest or drowning, the ability to pass a tracheal tube may be invaluable.

There are three essentials for the successful passage of a tube to the trachea:

1. Adequate relaxation of the muscles of the head, neck and larynx
2. Satisfactory positioning of the head and neck
3. The correct use of apparatus.

Anaesthesia for endotracheal intubation

Most commonly, the patient will have received an intravenous induction agent such as thiopentone which is followed immediately by the injection of a myoneural blocking drug such as suxamethonium. As soon as the myoneural block is established, the patient's lungs are ventilated with gas under pressure from a face piece and a reservoir bag and the patient is now ready for laryngoscopy and intubation. Alternatively, a deep level of anaesthesia may be induced with an inhalation anaesthetic such as halothane, or seroflurane to the point at which the cough reflex is obtunded. In these circumstances the conditions for laryngoscopy and intubation are obtained without the need for myoneural blockade.

The mouth, pharynx, laryngeal inlet and bronchial tree may be anaesthetized by the topical application of a local anaesthetic such as lignocaine from a metered dose aerosol. This technique is used when the induction of general anaesthesia as a preliminary to tracheal intubation may be fraught with danger because of difficulties in maintaining the airway, such as in patients with fixed deformities of the cervical spine.

In the resuscitation room it is common to find that the reasons demanding tracheal intubation are associated with unconsciousness, so that the question of anaesthesia does not arise.

Posture of the patient

The neck should be slightly flexed and the head extended. This has been described as a position for 'sniffing the air'. It is illustrated correctly in Figure 7.1 from which it can be seen that the correct position results in a straight line from the mouth through the vocal cords to the trachea. The common mistake is to extend the neck and the head as shown in Figure 7.2, and the resulting difficulties are obvious. It is often the case that when the head is correctly positioned in a patient whose muscles are sufficiently relaxed to allow tracheal intubation, the mouth will open slightly, allowing entry to the blade of the laryngoscope. Thus, the need to use one's fingers to open the mouth is a sign that the positioning is incorrect.

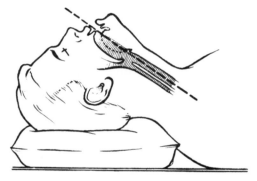

Fig. 7.1   Correct posture of head and neck for laryngoscopy. With the neck flexed and the head extended, the mouth, laryngoscope and trachea are in a straight line.

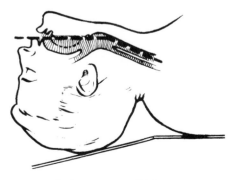

Fig. 7.2   Incorrect posture for laryngoscopy. With the neck and head extended, the trachea and laryngoscope blade are no longer in line.

Apparatus

The apparatus for direct or blind intubation of the trachea consists of laryngoscopes, tracheal tubes, aids to the introduction of the tracheal tube such as a malleable stilette, sprays for producing local analgesia of the larynx, and connectors to connect the tracheal tube to the anaesthetic apparatus or ventilator.

Laryngoscopes

Laryngoscopes may be divided into two groups: those with straight blades and those with curved blades. The first, typified by the Magill laryngoscope shown in Figure 7.3, is passed over the base of the tongue and the posterior surface of the epiglottis, exposing the larynx in a straight line. As the posterior surface of the epiglottis is supplied by the vagus nerve, reflexes set up by the use of this instrument tend to cause laryngeal spasm, and a deep level of general anaesthesia will be required to avoid this. The Macintosh laryngoscope (Fig. 7.4) was designed to pass over the base of the tongue but into the vallecula anterior to the epiglottis, an area which is supplied by the glossopharyngeal nerve. Figures 7.5 and 7.6 show the two instruments in use and illustrate this point. The use of the myoneural blocking drugs as an aid to laryngoscopy has lessened the need for the straight blade laryngoscope and the

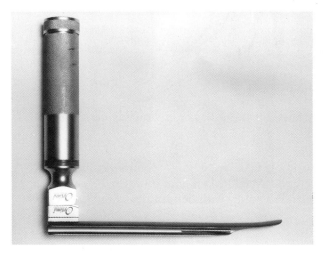

Fig. 7.3 Magill laryngoscope.

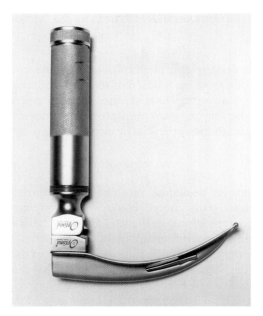

Fig. 7.4 Macintosh laryngoscope.

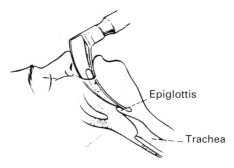

Epiglottis

Trachea

Fig. 7.5 Macintosh laryngoscope in use. The blade tip is anterior to the epiglottis.

Macintosh blade is used most commonly in modern practice. However, the Magill blade continues to be of use in paediatric practice and in adults with deformities of the jaw or neck.

Endotracheal tubes

These vary considerably in design. The commonest example

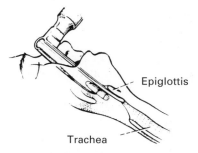

Fig. 7.6   Magill laryngoscope in use. The blade tip is posterior to the epiglottis.

(Fig. 7.7) is a curved tube with an angled aperture for insertion to the trachea and a cuff which is fixed to the outer surface of the tube near its distal end. The cuff may be inflated with air to provide a seal between the outer part of the tube and the lining of the trachea. A small indicator balloon on the inflation catheter of the cuff serves to reassure the anaesthetist that the cuff is functioning adequately. Sometimes it is preferable to have a tube without a cuff; such 'plain' tubes may be used for insertion through the nose (nasotracheal intubation) or may be preferred in circumstances in which the trachea is particularly at risk from pressure, such as might result from inflation of a cuff.

In certain circumstances, such as operations in which the position of the head may be changed several times during surgery, for example neurosurgery, or in operations in which a gag is placed in the mouth and may obstruct the tracheal tube, such as in procedures for the repair of a cleft palate or in tonsillectomy, reinforcement of the side of the tube may be required to prevent kinking or

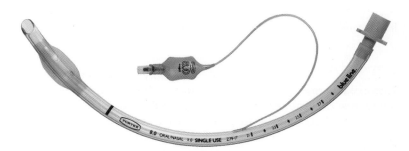

Fig. 7.7   Cuffed 'Portex' tube.

compression. Various forms of reinforced tubes are available. In some cases a nylon spiral may be used to reinforce the wall of the tube, while an alternative is the use of a tapered tube, the narrow distal end being of a size suitable for insertion to the larynx, while the more proximal part (in relation to the anaesthetist) is constructed of thick plastic or rubber which is less compressible than is the more commonly used tube. In the past, the majority of the commonly used tracheal tubes were made of red rubber and were re-used many times. This had the disadvantage of the high cost and difficulty of sterilization together with the risk of damage of the inflatable cuff when present. In most hospitals nowadays, tubes are made of plastic materials and are prepacked and sterilized by the manufacturer with the intention that they be discarded after use.

Intubating forceps (Fig. 7.8)

The example shown in Figure 7.8, designed by Magill, is in common use. The instrument is of great value during nasotracheal intubation in allowing the anaesthetist to manipulate the tip of the tube to the laryngeal inlet. These forceps are also of value when it is necessary to insert a nasogastric tube after anaesthesia has been induced.

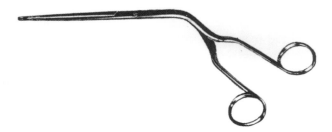

Fig. 7.8   Magill intubating forceps, curved to allow their use in the mouth, are used to guide an endotracheal tube through the vocal cords.

Laryngeal sprays

Laryngeal sprays have been designed to facilitate the deposition of a fine mist of local analgesic solution on the mucosa of the respiratory tract. This may be desirable even when general anaesthesia has been employed so that the reflexes caused by a tube as it passes into the trachea may be minimized. Figure 7.9 shows a commercial aerosol for lignocaine.

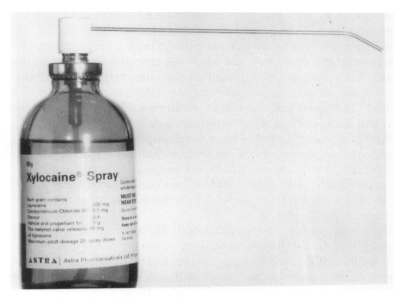

Fig. 7.9   Xylocaine (lignocaine) spray for topical use. Each spray action delivers 10 mg of drug. The maximum dose for a fit adult (200 mg) is 20 spray doses. The nozzle can be steam sterilized.

Connectors

The prepacked plastic tubes have a plastic connector included in the package. Such a connector is simple in design and allows easy access for suction catheters. There are various modifications of connectors which allow sampling of respired gas for monitoring.

It is important to ensure that the endotracheal tube and its connector are of such diameter that the resistance to flow through them is not excessive. It is also important to note that it is the narrowest part of the system that determines the magnitude of the resistance, so it is unwise to insert a connector to a tube unless it is of virtually the same diameter as the tube itself.

The technique of endotracheal intubation

Before commencing, it is important that everything should be at hand so that there is no delay once the procedure has started. The chosen laryngoscope should be tested to ensure that the light housed in the blade is working satisfactorily. It is particularly important to check that there is a suitable means of connecting the tracheal tube to the anaesthetic circuit or source of positive pressure ventilation. The internal diameter of the tube is given in millimetres on the outer wall and when the anaesthetist speaks of the 'size' of the tube it is this dimension that is referred to. The appropriate size of the tube is based on the patient's age in the case of a child. The age in years should be divided by four and 4.5 is added to the answer. Thus a 6.5 mm tube would be appropriate for a child of 8 years. However, there are considerable variations in the size of the larynx and many anaesthetists may wish to have in addition tubes which are one size bigger and one size smaller than the predicted tube. For adult patients, the tube sizes ranging from 8.0 mm (for a small woman) to 10.0 mm (for a large man) are appropriate.

A rough guide to the correct length of tube can be obtained by measuring the distance from the lobe of the ear to the angle of the mouth for oral intubation, or to the angle of the nose for nasal intubation. A tube cut to twice this length should reach from the incisor teeth or nostril to the midpoint of the trachea.

The laryngoscope is introduced into the patient's mouth along the right border of the tongue. The blade is slipped over the tongue until the epiglottis is visible. If a Magill laryngoscope is being used the epiglottis is lifted forward, whereas if a Macintosh laryngoscope is used the tip of the laryngoscope is inserted into the vallecula and the base of the tongue is lifted forward, carrying the epiglottis with it. A view such as that shown in Figure 7.10 will be obtained. The novice is often tempted to lever the handle of the laryngoscope to a more vertical position. Not only does this endanger the teeth but it will tend to push the larynx upwards and away from the field of vision.

Assuming that a good view of the laryngeal inlet has been obtained and that there is no danger of the inhalation of vomitus or blood at the end of the operation, one may decide to spray the vocal cords, and through the cords into the trachea, with a local anaesthetic. Similar qualifications apply to the use of local anaesthetic lubricants applied to the tube before insertion in the trachea. In patients who are undergoing surgery for the relief of intestinal obstruction, or operations on the mouth, throat or nose where blood may be present in the pharynx at the end of operation, a non-anaesthetic lubricant such as 'KY' jelly is preferred.

Where appropriate, the cuff of the tube is inflated with air at the same time as attempts are made to ventilate the lungs from a reser-

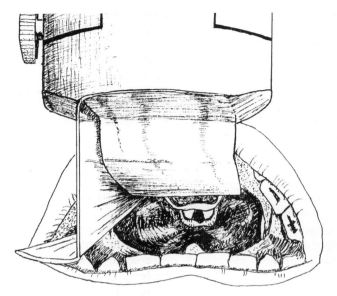

Fig. 7.10   View of the larynx and trachea obtained on direct laryngoscopy.

voir bag. The amount of air injected to the cuff should be just enough to prevent the audible return of the ventilating gas between the tube and the trachea.

Sometimes the nasotracheal route is used for securing an endotracheal airway. In cases in which direct laryngoscopy may be difficult, because of some inability to open the mouth or obtain access with the laryngoscope blade, there may be a case for passing the nasotracheal tube 'blindly', either with the patient conscious or under anaesthesia. Fibreoptic laryngoscopes have been designed as an aid in this type of manoeuvre, but considerable skill and experience are needed to use them safely in the difficult case.

Complications of endotracheal intubation

If there is difficulty in ventilating the patient's lungs, obstruction of the tube should be considered. The diagnosis can be confirmed by passing a finger into the mouth along the length of the tube. Kinking may be abolished by correct positioning of the head, and sometimes the introduction of an oropharyngeal airway into the mouth will help to prevent kinking. Occasionally, an excessively long tube may have been passed into the right bronchus. As a check against this possibility, it is essential to ensure that both lungs can be inflated. If necessary, this should be checked by auscultation.

Sore throat is common following endotracheal anaesthesia and probably occurs in about 50% of all patients at risk. The incidence may be reduced by care during the introduction of the tube and the use of adequate lubrication. The use of gauze packs to absorb blood, during tonsillectomy for example, is an additional factor which predisposes to sore throat in the postoperative period. This minor but nevertheless annoying complication can be treated if necessary with mild analgesics and mouthwashes.

Oedema of the larynx leads to laryngeal stridor and partial or complete obstruction of the airway. It is a rare complication of tracheal intubation in adults, but occurs more commonly in children. The treatment includes the inhalation of humidified oxygen or menthol vapour. In severe cases, helium–oxygen mixtures may be used and tracheostomy may be necessary if these simple measures fail. Laryngeal granulomata and tracheal stenosis are serious complications of tracheal intubation, but are associated more commonly with prolonged intubation such as might be necessary in the intensive therapy unit.

Difficult intubation

This is a widely recognized generic term for conditions in which orotracheal intubation as already described is either not easy or at times impossible. In some patients the anatomy of the mouth and pharynx is normal but a clear view of the epiglottis and laryngeal inlet is denied. Figure 7.11 shows the basis of a scoring system for recording the degree of difficulty.

In some patients the position of teeth can be a problem. Protruding upper teeth and incomplete dentition may obscure the view of the larynx. Some of the more difficult problems, however, stem from disease or injury ranging from severe displacement of the laryngeal inlet, for example as a result of thyroid enlargement, immobility of the neck as a result of spondylitis or fracture, 'floating' segments of the mandible or maxilla or oedema of the soft tissue of the mouth, or a combination of these, following injury. Grossly obese patients, particularly women, with a short neck may have a distribution of fat that prevents proper positioning of the laryngoscope handle and thus the blade.

In some patients difficulty with tracheal intubation is predictable

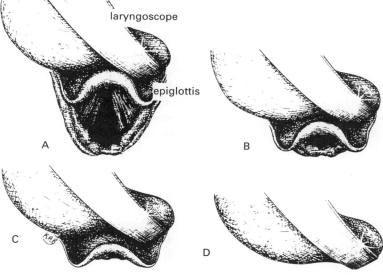

laryngoscope

epiglottis

A

B

C

D

Fig. 7.11   A–D show increasingly poor results of attempts to visualize the laryngeal inlet at laryngoscopy.

but in others it is completely unexpected. It is always important to know about difficulty in previous anaesthetics. The greatest anxiety for the safety of the patient occurs in the emergency case where the regurgitation of gastric contents in a patient whose airway is difficult to control could prove fatal.

There is a variety of strategies for dealing with difficult intubation. Sometimes it may be safe to abandon a decision to intubate, particularly as crude unsuccessful attempts at laryngoscopy can lead to oral or pharyngeal bleeding or oedema which can make the airway problem worse. Sometimes the use of a straight blade (Magill) laryngoscope can offer easier conditions than the Macintosh instrument. A malleable introducer inserted to the lumen of the tube may allow its curvature to be altered to make tracheal placement easier. It may be possible to insert a tracheal tube via the nose in such a way that its curvature allows 'blind' insertion to the trachea without the need for a laryngoscope. The development of fibreoptic laryngoscopes (Fig. 7.12) has saved the day in many cases by allowing the manipulation of a nasotracheal

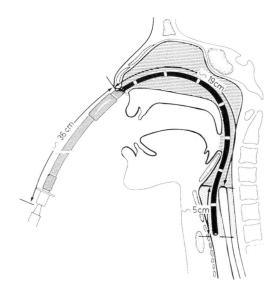

Fig. 7.12 Fibreoptic laryngoscopy.

tube to the correct position under direct vision. When special methods like these are used there is no substitute for skill and experience on the part of the anaesthetist. In many cases it is safer for these procedures to be conducted under topical anaesthesia of the upper airway, since general anaesthesia may be difficult to maintain and the presence of neuromuscular block may prove to be highly dangerous, since controlled ventilation of the lungs may be difficult to ensure.

Checking that the tracheal tube has been placed correctly

Serious brain injury or death result from unrecognized misplacement of a tracheal tube to the oesophagus instead of to the larynx. Thus as soon as the tube is thought to have been placed correctly its position can be verified by:

- Observing that the tip of the tube has entered the larynx
- Ventilating via the tube and listening to the movement of air within the lungs
- Listening with the stethoscope over the stomach to exclude the gurgling noises of misplaced ventilatory attempts to the oesophagus

- Monitoring the respired gas with a carbon dioxide analyser to determine that inspired gas contains practically no CO_2 but the end tidal expiration contains, as a rule, about 5% CO_2.

It is accepted in modern practice that in the absence of a CO_2 monitor there is no absolute guarantee of correct tracheal tube placement. This does not deny the fact that misdirection of ventilating gas to the oesophagus will ultimately be associated with signs of developing hypoxaemia and hypoxia, including cyanosis, desaturation as monitored by pulse oximeter, tachycardia, sweating and hypertension.

SPECIAL TUBES AND BLOCKERS

We have considered endotracheal tubes which are normally passed to a point midway between the cords and the bifurcation of the trachea. However, more elaborate tubes are available for the special needs of thoracic surgery. Depending on the particular design, these may be passed into one or other main bronchus so that the anaesthetic may be maintained via one lung while the other lung is allowed to collapse during the operation. These endobronchial tubes are narrower in diameter than are the endotracheal tubes and the design of the cuffs is critical so as to avoid obstruction of the lobar bronchi.

The administration of an anaesthetic into one lung is of particular value when the other lung is to be removed, and there are occasions when the anaesthetist may wish to inflate the lungs independently of one another. For this purpose, double lumen tubes, for example the Carlens tube (Fig. 7.13) or Robertshaw's tube, may be used.

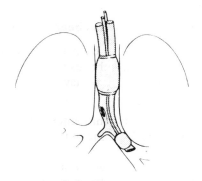

Fig. 7.13   Carlens double lumen tube. One or other lung can be ventilated independently.

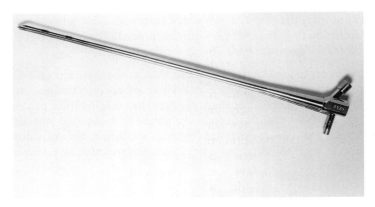

Fig. 7.14   Rigid bronchoscope for emergency use.

BRONCHOSCOPY

The indications for bronchoscopy in anaesthetic practice are the removal of secretions from the tracheobronchial tree and the removal of foreign bodies from the lungs. One may use a rigid bronchoscope as illustrated in Figure 7.14. There is a small light bulb at the distal end of the lumen.

The initial position of the patient's head for bronchoscopy is the same as for laryngoscopy, but thereafter the position must be altered so that the bronchoscope passes readily down the trachea to enter the main bronchi in correct alignment. This involves considerable repositioning of the head and the help of an assistant should be available.

There is a variety of techniques of anaesthesia for bronchoscopy. Topical (local) anaesthesia may be given without rendering the patient unconscious. A general anaesthetic may be induced with a non-flammable agent such as halothane and the patient is allowed to breathe spontaneously throughout. An alternative is to induce anaesthesia with an intravenous induction agent and thereafter to administer a short-acting myoneural blocking drug such as suxamethonium. Ventilation of the lungs may be continued with a suitable mixture of nitrous oxide and halothane in oxygen admitted through a side arm to the bronchoscope, with intermittent occlusion of the promixal end of the instrument to allow inflation of the lungs. Alternatively, a high-pressure injector device may be inserted to the lumen of the bronchoscope to admit oxygen through a venturi device with entrainment of room air in addition. The patient continues to be anaesthetized with intermittent injections of an intravenous anaesthetic, and supplementary injections of suxamethonium may be given if required.

Fibreoptic technology has revolutionized the methods for bronchoscopy, and increasingly fibreoptic bronchoscopes are preferred to rigid bronchoscopes for some problems described here. One of the many benefits of fibreoptic bronchoscopy is that the patient can breathe an anaesthetic mixture spontaneously. Although fibreoptic bronchoscopes have suction catheters built into the assembly, they may not be wide enough to cope with copious or viscid secretions, nor is the fibreoptic device appropriate for the removal of large particulate matter; for these purposes the rigid bronchoscope may be preferred.

Laryngeal mask airway

This device (Fig. 7.15) was introduced in the early 1980s and has gained wide acceptance. One end of the tube connects to the anaesthetic breathing system in a manner very similar to that for a tracheal tube. The other 'mask' end is positioned over the laryngeal inlet with an inflatable cuff around its aperture. It probably maintains the airway by keeping pharyngeal structures in position; but no one is sure of the mechanism. In many patients it enables the maintenance of a clear airway during spontaneous breathing in anaesthesia more easily than was possible traditionally, with or without an oropharyngeal Guedel-type device. In some patients artificial ventilation of the lungs may be achieved via a laryngeal mask airway but it is by no means reliable for this purpose and would not be regarded as a guaranteed solution to the problem of 'difficult' tracheal intubation (see above). The laryngeal mask offers no special protection to the lungs against the risk of accidental inspiration of gastric or other material from the pharynx.

The laryngeal mask airway is inserted blindly with the neck reasonably extended as in Figure 7.1; the mask with the cuff uninflated is passed with the curvature of the tube in line with the curvature of the tongue. Although the laryngeal mask can be inserted in patients who have received any of a variety of methods of general anaesthesia, the best conditions are achieved most rapidly following intravenous induction of anaesthesia with propofol and during the brief interval of respiratory depression which

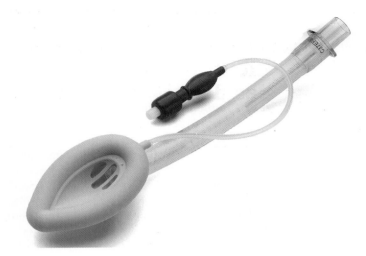

Fig. 7.15   Laryngeal mask airway.

may be associated with that. In contrast, attempts to perform the same manoeuvre following thiopentone instead of propofol are usually unsuccessful.

Sometimes the laryngeal mask may be an alternative to tracheal intubation in cardiopulmonary resuscitation.

8. The prevention and treatment of complications and difficulties during anaesthesia

In addition to watching for signs that the level of anaesthesia is adequate for the surgical operation, the anaesthetist must be prepared to anticipate and prevent, or diagnose and treat, several important complications; some are common, others are rare. Although some complications, such as vomiting and regurgitation, are characteristically associated with the induction of and recovery from anaesthesia, both these and other complications are risks associated with a light level of anaesthesia.

Accidental subcutaneous injection of intravenous anaesthetics

In the past there was much concern about accidental intra-arterial injection of thiopentone causing intimal damage and spasm of the vessel with ischaemia and death of tissue distal to the injection. The use of indwelling venous cannulae has almost removed this possible error. If it does occur there should be urgent treatment with vasodilators such as papaverine combined with immediate anticoagulant therapy with heparin 10 000 units i.v. followed by 5000 units given 6-hourly for 2 days. Sympathetic blockade by local anaesthetic infiltration around the stellate ganglion, or brachial plexus block, is also recommended.

Perivenous injection of thiopentone solution causes much discomfort and may risk tissue necrosis of the immediate area. Perivenous injection of methohexitone, etomidate or propofol is not associated with necrosis but can cause extreme discomfort, particularly if the volume injected is large.

Coughing

This is most likely to cause trouble during an attempted inhalation induction of anaesthesia. It may occur in response to material in the pharynx, such as mucus or even gastric contents, in which case, of course, it is a valuable protective reflex. Where it occurs in response to irritant vapours, notably ether and, to a lesser extent, isoflurane, it is still a demonstration of a protective reflex but is now an inconvenience since it delays the smooth uptake of the anaesthetic gas mixture to the lung. The remedy is to reduce the concentration of vapour and to consider the addition of a small quantity of carbon dioxide to the inspired gas. This will stimulate breathing and promote the uptake of the anaesthetic to the lung. Coughing may occur if an oropharyngeal airway or a laryngeal mask is inserted when the level of anaesthesia is too light; the recognition of this cause is usually obvious. On occasions, coughing may complicate the induction of anaesthesia with methohexitone or etomidate.

Breath-holding

Breath-holding can occur at a light level of anaesthesia and usually signifies that the patient is under the influence of a noxious stimulus to which he may be about to respond. Thus, breath-holding can be caused by irritant inhalation agents and may herald a bout of coughing. Alternatively, a patient who has apparently accepted an inhalation anaesthetic may breath-hold if an oropharyngeal airway is inserted at an unacceptably light level of anaesthesia. Again, coughing may be imminent. At a light level of anaesthesia, a powerful surgical stimulus, such as the incision of the skin or a stretching of the anal canal, may cause breath-holding following a deep inspiration. The addition of carbon dioxide to the inhaled mixture reduces the likelihood of breath-holding, although it is unlikely to be of much value once breath-holding has commenced. Other facets of management include withholding the surgical stimulus and reducing the concentration of the inhalation anaesthetic if this is thought to be irritating. The anaesthetist may be able to limit the period of breath-holding by partially closing the exhaust valve and applying gentle pressure to the anaesthetic reservoir bag, thus gently assisting the anaesthetic mixture towards the lungs. This technique demands experience and skill and we would not wish to give the impression that breath-holding is an indication for vigorous attempts at controlled ventilation. Breath-holding as described here must be distinguished from apnoea as a result of excessively deep anaesthesia or the effects of the myoneural blocking drugs. Making a differential diagnosis includes consideration of the period over which the patient has breathed the anaesthetic gas and the concentrations involved. In light anaesthesia such as would be associated with breath-holding, the respiratory effort up to the moment of cessation will have been vigorous; in these circumstances also, there may be considerable muscle tone, for example in the airway, while the eyelid reflex may be present or the eyes divergent. None of these signs is a feature of deep anaesthesia.

Airway obstruction

During anaesthesia, the airway may be obstructed for many reasons. The commonest is obstruction by the tongue when the muscles which are integrated into its substance lose their tone, thus enabling the tongue to fall towards the posterior wall of the pharynx in a patient who is lying in the supine position. This is accompanied by a noise similar to snoring. The problem is either treated or prevented by supporting the mandible as shown in Figures 8.1 and 8.2. Such correct positioning will prevent obstruction by the tongue in the majority of patients who have a well-formed mandible and good natural dentition. In the older patient whose mandible has been eroded by age and in all patients who have no teeth, these manoeuvres may not be sufficient on their own. It may be necessary to insert an oropharyngeal airway.

The upper airway may be obstructed by secretions or gastric contents in the pharynx and, in patients with head injuries, blood

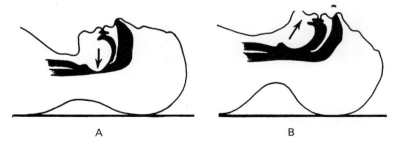

A   B

Fig. 8.1   These figures demonstrate the correct positioning of the head and jaw during anaesthesia and mouth-to-mouth breathing to ensure a clear airway. In A, the head is slightly flexed, the jaw is unsupported and the tongue has fallen back, obstructing the upper airway. In B, the head has been extended and the jaw pulled forward, taking the tongue with it and clearing the airway.

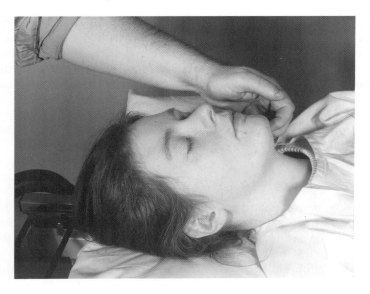

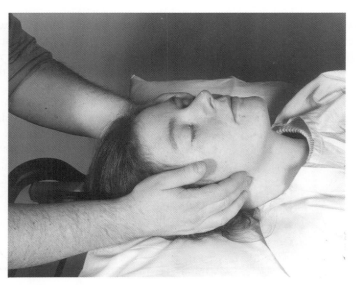

Fig. 8.2   Two alternative methods of supporting the unconscious patient's chin to prevent upper airway obstruction. Whether the tip of the chin or the angles of the jaw are supported, the direction of the pull is the same.

and cerebrospinal fluid may be present also. Various foreign bodies have been reported as causing obstruction of the upper airway, notably dentures.

The airway may be obstructed also by spasm of the larynx; other causes of laryngeal obstruction are oedema associated with acute infection, particularly in children, and tumours of the larynx or epiglottis. The trachea may be narrowed to the point of obstruction as a result of chondromalacia, or following prolonged external compression, for example by a tumour of the thyroid gland.

Laryngeal stridor and spasm

These are common and worrying causes of respiratory obstruction during light anaesthesia. Stridor is caused by an incomplete closure of the vocal cords during inspiration and is characterized by a high-pitched sound during inspiration. In laryngeal spasm the cords are closed completely; there is no noise because the obstruction is absolute. In both stridor and spasm there is usually exaggerated activity of the respiratory muscles. These complications may be a result of the irritation of the vocal cords by vapours, unwanted pharyngeal contents such as vomitus, or solid bodies such as an artificial airway. The ability to produce spasm of the cords is basically a protective reflex. Stridor and spasm may occur also as a result of impulses caused by events distant from the larynx, such as an incision of the skin or stretching of the anal sphincter.

Sometimes it is claimed that thiopentone, by heightening reflex excitability, may predispose to laryngeal spasm in the presence of irritants. Partial or complete closure of the laryngeal inlet causes hypoxia and retention of carbon dioxide. It is claimed that in healthy patients laryngeal spasm will always 'break' before death ensues because, as the patient becomes grossly hypoxic, the laryngeal muscles weaken and the larynx relaxes. It is unwise to depend on such assumptions, however. In any case, patients who are gravely ill will be placed at serious risk from a prolonged period of laryngeal spasm.

As a first stage in treatment, the source of any irritation should be withdrawn if possible. Thus, if a high concentration of an irritant anaesthetic is being administered, this should be reduced; if an airway has been inserted, this should be withdrawn partially. If it is suspected that fluid has accumulated in the pharynx, the patient's head should be lowered and suction applied to the pharynx. If the stimulus is from the surgical procedure, the surgeon should be asked to wait until the level of anaesthesia has been deepened.

If the closure of the larynx is only partial — that is, stridor is present — a high concentration of oxygen should be administered. The particular value of such therapy lies in the fact that reflex spasm is more likely to occur in the presence of hypoxia. If spasm is complete, gentle pressure on the reservoir bag with the exhaust valve almost closed and the circuit filled with oxygen is applied in the hope that the cords will relax momentarily, allowing oxygen to pass to the trachea and lungs. Of course, it is essential during these manoeuvres to ensure that the airway above the larynx is clear. If the spasm does not respond to these measures, the anaesthetist will normally administer a short-acting neuromuscular blocking drug such as suxamethonium 50 mg i.v. This will produce complete muscle relaxation and immediate separation of the cords. It is, of course, essential to control ventilation under these circumstances, and in most cases it would be appropriate to insert a tracheal tube. Meanwhile, suitable steps should be taken to deepen the level of anaesthesia.

Probably most of the deaths which have occurred as a result of laryngeal spasm could have been prevented if the anaesthetist had followed the simple guidance given above. Death from laryngeal spasm is unlikely to occur in experienced hands.

Rarely, if a neuromuscular blocking drug is not available and attempts to oxygenate the lungs have failed, a wide-bore needle should be inserted into the trachea through the midline at the midpoint of the cricothyroid membrane. A spontaneously breathing patient will be just able to ventilate the lungs through this narrow channel, and oxygen can be added to the air around the hub of the needle. Tracheotomy with a knife is neither necessary nor desirable in the treatment of this complication.

Bronchospasm

Occurring during anaesthesia, this may be mild, associated with a respiratory wheeze, or severe, in which case there may be no appreciable movement of air into and out of the lung, and the patient becomes cyanosed very rapidly. There are many causes of bronchospasm, including stimulation of the upper part of the respiratory tract at a light level of anaesthesia, for example by a tube in the trachea. Bronchospasm may be induced also by the presence of mucus in the respiratory tract. It is claimed that premedication with atropine not only reduces the likelihood of secretions but dilates the bronchial tree also.

Bronchospasm may occur as a result of histamine release following the injection of any one of a number of drugs during anaesthesia. It is probably true to say that few of the drugs given by intravenous injection during anaesthesia are free from risk of such reactions. Tubocurarine and morphine have a particular reputation in this respect.

A most worrying cause of bronchospasm during anaesthesia is the inhalation of gastric contents (Mendelson's syndrome). This condition is characterized by severe bronchospasm, pulmonary oedema and circulatory failure. The treatment of Mendelson's syndrome is detailed on page 129. Bronchospasm as a result of stimulation of the airway may be helped by the administration of aminophylline 250 mg i.v. and the instillation of 3 ml of 4% lignocaine via the endotracheal tube or by direct injection through the cricothyroid membrane. Adrenaline 0.2–0.4 mg i.v. for an adult, chlorpheniramine maleate (Piriton) 10 mg and hydrocortisone 100 mg are recommended in addition in cases of sensitivity to drugs. Because diethyl ether is a sympathetic stimulant, it has been suggested that controlled ventilation with about 5% of ether in the carrier gas will induce the bronchial musculature to relax. Above all, it is important to ensure that the patient receives a high concentration of oxygen in the inspired gas.

Hiccough

This may be very troublesome, particularly during abdominal surgery. It may be associated with the injection of methohexitone. The commonest cause, however, is surgical manipulation on the abdominal surface of the diaphragm. A reliable cure for this complication has still to be found, although asking the surgeon to reduce the level of stimulation is often successful. Hiccough may be an indication for deepening the level of anaesthesia, but it should not be regarded as an indication for increasing the dose of a neuromuscular blocking drug. Indeed, to do so may result in an excessively profound and refractory paralysis at the end of the operation.

Masseter spasm

The masseter muscles are extremely powerful and may develop

intense spasm at a light level of anaesthesia, particularly during induction and recovery. This may limit the anaesthetist's access to the mouth and endanger life if there is a need to aspirate material from the pharynx. An additional difficulty arises if an orotracheal tube is in position, because the patient's teeth may obstruct the tube totally. Although masseter spasm will disappear spontaneously as the level of anaesthesia either lightens or deepens, it may be necessary to give a short-acting myoneural blocking drug to enable the more severe difficulties associated with a masseter spasm to be avoided. On occasion, a gag such as that shown in Figure 8.3 may be used to force the mouth open; the danger of damage to the teeth from the inexperienced use of this device is considerable.

INADEQUATE VENTILATION

We have considered some of the more dramatic complications which may occur during general anaesthesia. However, equally important is the less dramatic occurrence of inadequate gas exchange which may occur during either spontaneous breathing or controlled ventilation. The problem can be considered under two headings: inadequacy of alveolar ventilation, and factors impeding oxygenation of the arterial blood.

Inadequacy of alveolar ventilation

In the spontaneously breathing anaesthetized patient, the commonest causes of under-ventilation are depression of the respiratory centres, which may occur at any stage during the anaesthetic, or partial neuromuscular block as a result of inadequate antagonism of myoneural blockade, occurring at the end of anaesthesia or in the early postoperative period. The ventilation may be inadequate

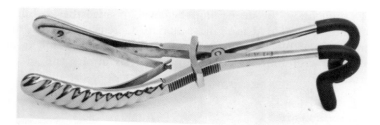

Fig. 8.3   Mouth gag.

in a patient who is undergoing controlled ventilation for which inadequate ventilating volumes have been provided.

For any particular patient there is a predictable relationship between the amount of the alveolar ventilation, and the alveolar and arterial carbon dioxide tension (PCO_2,). This relationship is shown in Figure 8.4; it can be seen that the average alveolar ventilation required to maintain the arterial PCO_2 at the normal value of 5.3 kPa is about 4 litre/min. Figure 8.4 shows also that under-ventilation leads to a rapid increase in the alveolar PCO_2, whereas excessive ventilation (such as may occur as a result of large tidal volumes during controlled ventilation) leads to a reduction in PCO_2.

Normally, when ventilation is reduced, carbon dioxide accumulates in the alveolar gas. The combination of a high alveolar carbon dioxide content and an inadequate supply of oxygen to the alveoli, because of under-ventilation, causes hypoxaemia to co-exist with hypercarbia. However, carbon dioxide may be retained without obvious signs of hypoxaemia if a high concentration of oxygen is given to the patient. This occurs particularly when oxygen is used as the sole carrier gas, for example in the administration of halothane-in-oxygen anaesthesia. It is particularly important to

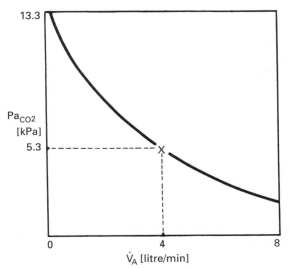

Fig. 8.4   This graph illustrates the relationship between alveolar ventilation ($\dot{V}_A$) and arterial carbon dioxide tension ($PaCO_2$).

appreciate this fact since the agents which are commonly given with oxygen as the sole carrier gas — halothane and sevoflurane, for example — are powerful respiratory depressants.

Inadequate ventilation may be detected by:

- *Direct measurement of the arterial P_{CO_2}.* This is the most reliable index.
- *Measurement of the respiratory minute volume.* This requires an instrument such as the Wright respirometer. In this case the patient's basal requirements may be obtained from tables. Alternatively, it may be reasonable to decide that the patient will not be allowed to develop a minute volume of less than 5 litre/min. It is important, of course, to remember that it is the *alveolar* minute volume which matters and that the respirometer allows us to measure only the alveolar ventilation and the dead-space ventilation combined.

The clinical signs of under-ventilation and carbon dioxide retention. These signs appear when the arterial P_{CO_2} has reached levels between 10 and 12 kPa and are as follows:

- A hot, flushed, moist skin — the so-called boiled lobster syndrome. This is caused by dilatation of the arterioles and capillaries by local action of carbon dioxide.
- The central action of carbon dioxide on the vasomotor centre results in vasoconstriction of the larger vessels, in particular the splanchnic vessels, which results in an increase in arterial pressure.
- The heart rate increases in the early stages of carbon dioxide-retention, although in the later stages the conducting mechanism of the heart is poisoned and the rate slows before the heart fails.
- The physiological respiratory response to carbon dioxide is an increase in the depth or rate of respiration, or both; but the anaesthetist must not depend too much on these signs since it is often in circumstances in which the patient cannot respond by increasing the rate or depth of respiration that carbon dioxide retention occurs.
- If the operation has started, there may be increased oozing from the skin edges.
- If carbon dioxide retention occurs when the patient is not anaesthetized, for example in the postoperative period, the patient may be seen to be restless and confused.

Reduced arterial P_{O_2}

This is most immediately detected by observing cyanosis of the lips and ears or a reduced saturation value from a pulse oximeter (Sp_{O_2}). The most serious problem of oxygenation occurs when the inspired oxygen concentration is less than that in ambient air. The most dramatic example is sudden failure of the oxygen supply to an anaesthetic circuit, with continued supply of nitrous oxide. Such gross asphyxia will lead to circulatory arrest within about 3 minutes.

A more subtle and less dramatic cause of hypoxaemia has been noted in Chapter 2. Under most circumstances of general anaesthesia, there is an increase in the amount of right-to-left shunt across the lung. This is a mixture of both true shunting through discrete nonventilated channels and a 'shunt-like' effect (an excess of perfusion in relation to ventilation, particularly in the dependent regions of the lung). For practical purposes the effects of these changes on the arterial P_{O_2} may be overcome by the administration of not less than 30–40% of oxygen in the inspired gas. However, this statement applies only to patients with normal or near normal cardiorespiratory function. In patients with cyanotic heart disease or with serious lung disease, the maintenance of adequate oxygenation during anaesthesia is one of the major challenges to the anaesthetist.

While it is now reognized that during spontaneous breathing with many of the volatile anaesthetics oxygen tensions below the ideal level and carbon dioxide tensions of almost twice normal have been reached and apparently tolerated by healthy individuals, early recognition of inadequate ventilation is desirable and should be an indication for assisted or controlled ventilation, or an increase in the inspired oxygen concentration as appropriate. Apart from the specific signs associated with hypoxaemia (cyanosis) and carbon dioxide retention (sweating, hypertension, etc.), it is important for all doctors to recognize the abnormal pattern of breathing which is often associated with early respiratory failure. The classic appearance is that of excessive use of the diaphragm in relation to the intercostal muscles. This causes a see-saw type of breathing in which the chest may be drawn in and the abdominal wall protruded during inspiration, and vice versa on expiration. Since a jerking movement of the diaphragm occurs also, there may be a tugging action on the mediastinal structures, seen most obviously as a 'tracheal tug'. This effect is most likely to be present in elderly subjects in whom the mediastinum is relatively rigid.

CIRCULATORY COMPLICATIONS

Complications affecting the circulation during anaesthesia may be considered in two main groups. These are: changes in arterial pressure, and changes in heart rate and rhythm.

Changes in arterial pressure

The pressure may decrease, increase or fluctuate widely.

Hypotension

Hypotension may be caused by a variety of factors during anaesthesia. Some of these are associated with central depression of the vasomotor centre, resulting in vasodilatation, some with depression of the myocardium, resulting in a decreased cardiac output, some with diminished venous return to the heart, and others with blood loss.

It is not unusual for a patient, having received premedication, to arrive at the anaesthetic room with an arterial systolic pressure of 25 mmHg, or more, less than the resting level as measured in the ward. This is not an unexpected phenomenon since arterial pressure may decrease by about that amount during normal sleep.

Occasionally, the decrease in pressure is more marked, particularly with some premedicants such as phenothiazine drugs and pethidine. On occasion, marked hypotension may indicate that the patient's functional extracellular fluid volume is abnormally low, such as may occur in hot conditions where there has been profuse sweating or in patients who have suffered peritonitis with considerable loss of fluid into the peritoneal cavity. The administration of thiopentone or propofol and many of the techniques which may be used for the maintenance of anaesthesia may cause mild hypotension, particularly before the surgical stimulus has been applied. After surgery has commenced, however, it is common to find the arterial pressure restored to a level not far removed from the resting value.

Prolonged marked hypotension carries the risk of cerebral and myocardial damage from hypoxia, or thrombus formation. The oxygenation of these and other tissues does not depend entirely on the level of the arterial pressure. The arterial oxygen content and the blood flow, which varies from organ to organ, and the pooling of blood in dependent parts are all important factors. A further complication, where low blood pressure persists for a long period, is that the renal and hepatic circulation may be inadequate, with consequent damage to these organs.

The critical mean arterial pressure below which such damage may occur is a matter of some doubt and must be considered in relation to the adequacy of the arterial oxygen availability, although it is widely recognized that renal damage may ensue when the mean pressure falls below 50 mmHg. The critical value may be less than this in some types of deliberately induced arterial hypotension, for example high spinal (subarachnoid) nerve block. However, unless the anaesthetist wishes to reduce the arterial pressure deliberately, it is regarded as good practice to maintain the mean pressure as close as possible to the normal resting value.

Treatment

- Where hypotension is thought to be the result of depression by drugs such as halothane, the concentration of the agent should be reduced if possible. As a safeguard, the concentration of oxygen in the inspired gas should be increased. If there is an associated bradycardia (pulse rate less than 55 per min), atropine 0.6 mg i.v. will increase the heart rate and the arterial pressure. An adrenergic stimulator such as ephedrine (3–5 mg i.v.) may be helpful.

- When ventilation is controlled artificially, the changes in intrathoracic pressure abolish the respiratory pump action (vis a fronte) which allows the heart and great veins to fill during inspiration. This potentially harmful effect of intermittent positive pressure ventilation is discussed more fully in Chapter 10. In general, however, it is wise to reduce the mean intrathoracic pressure to the lowest possible value consistent with adequate ventilation.

- Hypotension resulting from loss of blood or extracellular water should be treated by the infusion of blood, plasma, plasma substitutes or the appropriate electrolyte solution (see Ch. 5). Elevation of the legs is an important first aid measure.

Hypertension

When this occurs during anaesthesia, it may be a result of under-ventilation of the lungs with the retention of carbon dioxide and the development of hypoxaemia. The problem has been discussed earlier in this chapter. The treatment may involve the institution of controlled ventilation or an increase in the ventilating volumes, if ventilation is being controlled already.

Hypertension may also occur as a response to the surgical stimulus in a patient who has received inadequate amounts of analgesics. This can be confirmed by looking for other signs of reflex activity and by administering supplementary analgesia, either additional volatile agents to the anaesthetic gas mixture or the intravenous administration of a small dose of a narcotic analgesic.

A rare cause of severe hypertension during anaesthesia is the presence of a phaeochromocytoma.

Hypertension or hypotension are more marked in patients with pre-existing arterial hypertension and in those receiving β-blockers. Such patients are more susceptible to the cardiovascular effects of drugs, mechanical ventilation and blood loss. They may also show a marked hypertensive response to inadequate analgesia during surgery.

Changes in heart rate and rhythm

Tachycardia may follow the administration of some drugs used in anaesthesia. It may be a physiological response to hypotension or may be caused by drugs with vagolytic effects, such as atropine or pethidine. Tachycardia may be a sign of excessively light anaesthesia.

Whereas tachycardia as a result of the administration of drugs may be accepted, it should be remembered that it may also be associated with haemorrhage or inadequacy of analgesia or ventilation. In these circumstances it is a sign which calls for action to treat the underlying condition.

Bradycardia may occur in association with the administration of halothane and it is often advisable to give atropine as a premedicant before the use of these agents. Even if premedication with atropine has been given, the occurrence of severe bradycardia (pulse rate 55 per minute or less) during anaesthesia with these agents may call for the administration of additional atropine 0.3–0.6 mg. Bradycardia may also follow the administration of suxamethonium and may be profound, particularly after a second or subsequent dose. Again, this problem can be minimized by the prophylactic administration of atropine and by restricting the second and further doses of suxamethonium to a maximum of 25 mg.

Cardiac arrhythmias of various types occur during anaesthesia and are particularly associated with the administration of halogenated anaesthetics such as halothane. Many reasons have been advanced for their occurrence but it is now generally agreed that they occur principally when the arterial carbon dioxide tension is high during the administration of these agents. Although it has been shown that arrhythmias are present frequently without any great harm resulting, they should always be considered potentially dangerous, and adequate ventilation must be maintained. If this does not cause the arrhythmias to disappear, the concentration of the anaesthetic agent should be reduced or a change made to another agent. Nodal rhythm is a typical sign of excessively deep halothane anaesthesia. Ventricular extrasystole is a potentially serious arrhythmia which almost always indicates a need to reduce the concentration of any volatile hydrocarbon administered.

The arrhythmias may, of themselves, be a sign of severe carbon dioxide retention and lack of oxygen.

Where the heart beat is absent and a pulse cannot be felt in a major vessel such as the carotid, a provisional diagnosis of cardiac arrest should be made and confirmatory signs sought. It must be stressed that such a diagnosis is made only when pulsation in a major vessel cannot be felt and not when pulsation cannot be obtained in the radial or facial arteries, because pulsation in these vessels may be absent during anaesthesia for a variety of reasons, such as pressure of harnesses or vasoconstriction. When the carotid pulse is absent, the apex beat should be checked rapidly with a stethoscope or by palpation. The absence of a heart beat or of pulsation in the major vessel confirms the diagnosis of cardiac arrest.

At this point, a carefully organized plan must be put into effect because, within 3 or 4 minutes of cessation of circulation, irreparable damage to the brain will result. When cardiac massage is instituted, the anaesthetist should ensure that ventilation of the lungs with 100% oxygen is continued throughout the attempts at resuscitation. The problems of cardiac arrest and the methods of dealing with it are considered in greater detail in the section dealing with resuscitation (see Ch. 11).

Finger plethysmographs have the disadvantage that, during surgery, they tend to pick up extraneous movements of the limb to which they are attached, and during operations when vasoconstriction takes place, the record of each beat may be extremely faint. Nevertheless, awareness of vasoconstriction as a result of such findings is useful information in itself.

The uncertainty in interpreting central venous pressure measurement during operation is considered on page 236.

VOMITING AND REGURGITATION

These are particular hazards during induction and recovery, although regurgitation may occur at any time during the maintenance of anaesthesia also.

Vomiting is an active reflex activity involving integrated action of the respiratory muscles, the larynx and the vomiting and respiratory centres in the medulla. The process cannot occur unless there is such a degree of reflex integrity that the patient is conscious and the cough reflex is present. Thus, the risk to the respiratory tract is much less than in the case of regurgitation.

Regurgitation is the result of the intragastric pressure being sufficiently great to overcome the competence of the sphincter-like protective mechanisms at the lower end of the oesophagus. Thus, regurgitation can occur both in the enfeebled conscious patient and also in the unconscious, and it constitutes a serious risk that the regurgitated material will spill over into the respiratory tract.

The risk of vomiting and regurgitation is so great that anaesthesia should not be undertaken in a patient who is known to have food in the stomach unless the indications for operation are extremely urgent. The normal emptying time of the stomach is somewhere between 4 and 5 hours. This may be hastened by the use of a drug such as metoclopramide (Maxolon) 20 mg i.v., and may be delayed following the ingestion of a fatty meal or as a consequence of injury.

Various manoeuvres have been introduced to promote the emptying of the stomach before anaesthesia is undertaken in an emergency. These include the insertion of tubes for the aspiration of stomach contents or the administration of apomorphine to induce vomiting. Quite apart from the barbaric nature of these measures, they are unacceptable because they cannot be guaranteed to be effective.

The treatment of vomiting and regurgitation is to lower the patient's head and turn it to one side; the vomitus should be aspirated from the pharynx. During light anaesthesia this may be all that is required and, if the anaesthetic is continued with the head down and to the side, regurgitated material is unlikely to pass into the trachea. If inhalation of vomitus has taken place, steps should be taken to aspirate the tracheal contents immediately, either through an endotracheal tube or by bronchoscopy. The use of a head-down posture may assist these measures.

Sellick's manoeuvre. If an assistant applies firm pressure on the cricoid cartilage with the thumb and index finger (Fig. 8.5), this will occlude the oesophagus and is probably the most effective precaution which can be taken to prevent regurgitated stomach contents from reaching the laryngeal inlet.

The insertion of a cuffed tracheal tube as early as possible in the conduct of an anaesthetic will not prevent vomiting or regurgitation, but will play a major part in ensuring that the gastric contents do not reach the bronchial tree. It is foolish to assume, however, that cuffed tubes offer total protection; the cuff may rupture or its seal with the trachea may be inadequate.

If gastric contents enter the respiratory tract, attempts should be made to remove the material as rapidly as possible by suction with a fine catheter through a tracheal tube. If the quantity is considerable, or the pH of the contents irrespective of quantity is very low, there is a risk of the development of aspiration pneumonitis (Mendelson's syndrome), characterized by acute bronchospasm and circulatory collapse. The mortality from Mendelson's syndrome is difficult to measure but may amount to about 25% of all patients who develop the condition. The lungs should be ventilated artificially with oxygen-enriched air and antispasmodic agents such as aminophylline, antibiotics and hydrocortisone should be given intravenously. In addition, support of the circulation by the administration of plasma expanders is important.

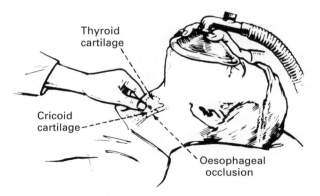

Thyroid cartilage

Cricoid cartilage

Oesophageal occlusion

Fig. 8.5   Firm pressure on the cricoid by an assistant during induction of anaesthesia may prevent regurgitation of stomach contents by occluding the oesophagus.

There is a serious risk of inhalation of blood to the lungs if this is present in the pharynx, for example after tonsillectomy.

MALIGNANT HYPERPYREXIA

This is the name given to a syndrome whose main features are increased muscle tone, high fever and a massive increase in the body's oxygen consumption. While it may occur in association with any inhalation anaesthetic, it is seen most often when suxamethonium or halothane has been used. The incidence varies in different populations but is quoted as 1 in 100 000 operations requiring anaesthetic. It is associated with an inherited abnormality which may be revealed by abnormal levels of the serum concentration of creatine phosphokinase (CPK) or by muscle biopsy. It is suggested that the condition may be associated with various myopathies which occasionally manifest themselves as an inguinal hernia or strabismus in a child.

Treatment is directed towards lowering the body temperature and correcting the metabolic acidosis and hyperkalaemia which develop. Dantrolene sodium is the drug of choice in the treatment of the condition. 1 mg/kg body weight is given and this can be repeated up to ten times if necessary over a period of about an hour. Dantrolene is a muscle relaxant (but not a neuromuscular blocker) which acts by modifying calcium release from the muscle cytoplasmic reticulum. The anaesthetic should be discontinued immediately and the lungs ventilated with 100% oxygen. Glucose in a 50% solution with insulin (100 units to 1 litre of infusion) is infused slowly and sodium bicarbonate is given to correct the metabolic acidosis which develops very rapidly. The patient's body is covered in ice packs or cooling lotions and the temperature must be monitored accurately.

Signs that treatment is effective include a reduction in body temperature and in the pressure that must be applied to ventilate the lungs artificially; the latter may become very high in view of the massive increase in muscle tone associated with the condition.

There is a high mortality from malignant hyperpyrexia and relatives of susceptible patients should be screened with a view to preventing a similar occurrence at a later date. There have been tragic examples of two mishaps in one family because such precautions were not taken. Careful interpretation of CPK values with biochemical advice, perhaps muscle biopsy for in vitro examination of the effects of various anaesthetics on the muscle specimen, and correlation with previous anaesthetic experiences are advised.

Any subsequent operations upon survivors or their families should be conducted under general anaesthesia, in which thiopentone, the non-depolarizing myoneural blocking drugs, oxygen, nitrous oxide and narcotic analgesics such as morphine or phenoperidine are the only agents which are completely safe. In spite of this, there is one report of malignant hyperpyrexia having been triggered by exposure to nitrous oxide. It should be emphasized that susceptibility to malignant hyperpyrexia is a contraindication to the use of local anaesthetic drugs, especially lignocaine, which are thought to be able to trigger the condition also.

9. Recovery room: postoperative care of patients

All patiens should be observed during the postoperative period in a centralized recovery room beside the operating theatre. The length of stay in this room will depend on the condition of the patient and the nature of the surgical procedure and anaesthesia. It is essential that all nurses and medical staff engaged in postoperative care should be trained specially for this work and should be capable of carrying out certain emergency resuscitative measures.

In the UK the concept of a postoperative recovery room was almost universally accepted by the late 1970s. The progress of a patient might be from recovery room to surgical ward or, in the case of the seriously ill, via the intensive care unit and then to the surgical ward. Because of the inability of surgical wards to cope with the increasing technology of the postoperative period at the level of electronic monitoring, syringe drivers etc., the desirability of an additional postoperative care area called the High Dependency Unit, in which a patient might remain for 24 hours or more, became increasingly recognized. Nowadays some health care experts consider that the concept of *progressive patient care* is inevitable. Thus, in addition to the stages of care that we have mentioned, some patients who need to reside for a time near the hospital, but are not in need of any nursing or therapeutic inter-vention, might be more efficiently cared for in an *hotel* facility.

COMPLICATIONS OF ANAESTHESIA

There are five groups of complications which may require the spe-cial attention of recovery room staff:

- *Respiratory*: obstruction of the airway; respiratory inadequacy and respiratory arrest
- *Circulatory*: hypotension; cardiac irregularities and cardiac arrest
- *Gastrointestinal*: vomiting or regurgitation of stomach contents

133

- *Renal*: acute reversible renal failure
- *Neurological sequelae.*

These main groups may frequently overlap; for example, a patient while still recovering from anaesthesia may regurgitate, inhale gastric contents and suffer respiratory obstruction. Untreated, this could lead to cardiac arrest and death.

We will now consider these complications in more detail, describing their mechanism, recognition and appropriate treatment.

Respiratory complications

Obstruction of the airway

The commonest respiratory complication in the immediate post-operative period is obstruction of the patient's upper airway. The three commonest causes are: the tongue falling back against the posterior wall of the pharynx when the patient is supine; the presence of foreign material in the pharynx, notably blood in patients undergoing tonsillectomy and other operations in the mouth, nose or pharynx; and laryngeal spasm. Respiratory obstruction can be diagnosed when movements of the chest and abdomen are exaggerated, but very little air passes through the nose or mouth, with the patient becoming increasingly cyanosed. Laryngeal spasm often produces a 'crowing' noise as air passes through the constricted larynx. It is worth remembering that *noisy breathing is always obstructed breathing, but not all obstructed breathing is noisy.*

Treatment. Secure a clear airway immediately. This is usually accomplished by pulling the lower jaw upwards and forwards, thus pulling the tongue away from the posterior pharyngeal wall. An oropharyngeal airway should be inserted if the patient will tolerate it. The patient should be placed in the lateral position and this may in itself improve the airway. If laryngeal spasm is the cause of the problem, suxamethonium may have to be given followed by a period of artificial ventilation of the lungs. Suction may be required to remove any obstruction, for example mucus. As a rule, oxygen should be administered, but it is quite useless to do this alone unless the airway is clear.

If no improvement follows simple manoeuvres, the relatively inexperienced should *summon help* quickly. This advice is particularly relevant if suxamethonium has to be given with a view to re-intubation of the trachea, etc.

Respiratory insufficiency

Despite an unobstructed upper airway, some patients may not breathe deeply enough to ensure adequate respiratory exchange in the alveoli. Any interference with this mechanism results in hypoxia and carbon dioxide accumulation (Figs 8.4, 9.1). This may occur for many reasons:

Obstruction of the smaller airways or bronchoconstriction
Depression of the respiratory centre following head injuries or cerebrovascular accidents, or the prolonged effects of anaesthetic agents
Disease of or damage to the nervous pathways to the muscles of respiration, for example peripheral neuropathy, poliomyelitis

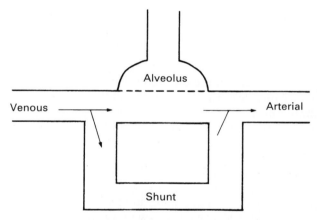

Fig. 9.1   Diagram showing alveolus of a healthy patient in contact with pulmonary capillary blood flow. Some of the venous blood reaching the alveoli in the pulmonary artery is shunted away from the alveolar exchange and renders the arterial gas tensions different from those of blood which has achieved total equilibrium with alveolar gas. Gas tension is in kPa. It is assumed that the patient is breathing air and that the haemoglobin concentration is 14.8 g/dl.

	P_{O_2}	P_{CO_2}	O_2 content (ml)	% saturation	CO_2 content (ml)
Venous blood	5.3	6.1	14.9	75	52
Blood exchanging with alveolus	13.7	5.3	19.7	98	47.5
Shunt	5.3	6.1	14.9	75	52
Arterial blood	12.4	5.4	19.6	97	48
Alveolar gas	13.7	5.3	—	—	—

Weakness of the muscles of respiration, as in myasthenia gravis, or when the action of relaxant drugs has not been fully reversed at the end of the operation
Removal of lung tissue, as in lobectomy or pneumonectomy
Pre-existing lung disease, for example bronchitis or emphysema
Interference with normal expansion of the lung during breathing. This may be the result of pre-existing disease of the thoracic cage, for example ankylosing spondylitis, or trauma to the chest wall with fractured ribs. A simpler cause sometimes found is the application of a tight dressing following operation or severe pressure on the undersurface of the diaphragm, such as may follow repair of a large ventral hernia. The recognition of inadequate respiration has already been discussed (p. 123).

If the patient has previously been conscious, respiratory inadequacy may be evidenced by increasing restlessness, confusion, drowsiness and eventual coma.

Treatment. Having secured a clear airway, the next step, no matter what the underlying cause of the respiratory inadequacy, must always be to assist the patient's own inadequate efforts. Increasing the amount of oxygen in the inspired air alone, although a reasonable first aid measure, rarely results in permanent improvement. Many simple devices are now available to augment the patient's ventilation. These enable the doctor or nurse to administer atmospheric air enriched with oxygen by intermittent compression of a bag or bellows, for example the Ambu resuscitator (Fig. 9.2).

No recovery room should be without one of these simple devices and all staff should be skilled in their use. When apparatus is not immediately available, the physician must resort to other measures to support the patient's failing or absent ventilation. The simplest and most effective of these measures is the technique of expired air resuscitation or mouth-to-mouth breathing. A detailed description of this method is given in Chapter 11.

Circulatory complications

When considering *circulatory changes* following anaesthesia, it is important to remember the significance of alterations in the patient's colour. Pallor or flushing in the absence of other signs of shock or inadequate respiration may be quite normal. Cyanosis *always* calls for urgent treatment.

The temperature of patients returning to a recovery room may

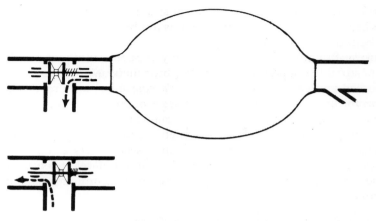

Fig. 9.2   Ambu resuscitator: additional oxygen may be fed into the bag through the small side tube at the right of the picture, thus enriching the air which is driven into the patient's lungs when the bag is compressed. On the left of the illustration is the non-return valve connected to a mask or endotracheal tube by the vertical limb. The patient's expirations are delivered to the atmosphere through the horizontal limb of the valve.

often be found to be slightly subnormal. While it is important to prevent such patients from shivering, only exceptionally should heat be applied, as this results in diversion of the blood from the vital organs to the skin.

Pulse

The pulse rate should be observed carefully during the immediate postoperative period.

A moderate tachycardia (80–100 beats/min) commonly follows major surgery, but a persistent tachycardia, particularly if it is increasing, should always be regarded as a danger sign, indicating perhaps haemorrhage or inadequate respiration.

Arterial pressure

Following a major operation the arterial pressure may be below the preoperative value as a result of the surgery itself and the continuing action of drugs administered by the anaesthetist. A systolic pressure of about 20 mmHg below the preoperative value can often be accepted, but where it continues to increase or decrease unduly an explanation should be sought. All patients who have had a general anaesthetic, and some to whom a regional analgesic has been given, are liable to hypotension and even sudden cardiac arrest if they are roughly handled or put in the sitting-up position (postural hypotension); they should be moved gently from trolley to bed and kept flat (or in the tonsillar position) until recovery is complete. In some circumstances the bed may be tilted to a moderate (5–10°) head-down position for the first hour or two.

Frequent arterial pressure readings are time consuming and not usually necessary (for example, not in excess of every 15 minutes). Close observation of colour change in the skin, level of consciousness and pulse rate provides the necessary information in most patients.

There are some patients for whom continuous arterial pressure recording during anaesthesia and throughout the recovery period is necessary. This is common after major cardiothoracic procedures or following surgery and anaesthesia in patients with severe multiple injuries. Accurate and continuous measurement of arterial pressure is achieved in this situation by means of an indwelling arterial cannula coupled to a pressure transducer system, with the resulting signal displayed on an oscilloscope, analogue or digital meter, or recorder.

Venous pressure

Where central venous pressure has been measured during anaesthesia, measurements may continue to be made during the recovery period as a guide to further blood or plasma requirements. In certain circumstances measurement of central venous pressure can be misleading because of previous cardiac or pulmonary disease, and pressure recordings from the left side of the heart more truly reflect the performance of the heart as a pump. In special cases (usually major cardiovascular surgery) it may be desirable to pass a flow-directed catheter (Swan–Ganz type) via the superior vena cava through the right atrium and ventricle and allow it to wedge in a branch of the pulmonary artery. These catheters have a number of functions. The pulmonary wedge pressure is nearly identical to the left atrial pressure and changes in its value can provide a more precise guide for the clinician as to the need for further intravenous infusions or the administration of cardiac inotropic drugs such as isoprenaline when there is evidence of a failing heart. A catheter also allows measurement of pulmonary artery pressure and the injection of liquids into the pulmonary artery. Some types of catheter have a heat sensitive probe incorporated so that the injection of saline at room temperature to the pulmonary artery will allow a thermodilution method for estimation of the cardiac output.

Cardiac arrest

Cardiac irregularities in the postoperative period should always be reported to the anaesthetist. Atrial fibrillation in elderly patients may occur following major surgery, and its onset is often accompanied by a fall in blood pressure. Bursts of extrasystoles (dropped beats) may herald the onset of ventricular fibrillation and cardiac arrest. The precise diagnosis of cardiac irregularities usually depends on the ECG, and therefore the earlier their occurrence is reported the better.

The most sudden and dramatic of all emergencies with which the recovery room personnel may have to deal is that of cardiac arrest. This may follow untreated respiratory inadequacy or a period of persistent hypotension due to any cause, but it can frequently occur without warning. Any patients who are especially at risk, for example those with some degree of heart-block preoperatively, should be indicated to the staff by the anaesthetist. Even in previously healthy adults, the sensitive tissue of the brain will only survive the results of circulatory standstill and acute hypoxia for a period of about 3 minutes. The immediate recognition of this condition is therefore of the utmost importance if resuscitation is to be successful.

Signs of 'apparent cardiac arrest'. The term 'apparent cardiac arrest' is used deliberately since, if the cardiac action and circulation are so poor that the following signs are present, then immediate treatment is required even if the heart has not quite stopped. There are three signs:

- *Pallor or cyanosis of the skin,* that is, a sudden deterioration of the skin colour.
- *Absence of palpable carotid pulses in the neck*; NB: not the radial pulses as these are often difficult to feel.
- *Rapidly dilating pupils.* This is the most reliable sign of cerebral hypoxia.

Two secondary signs should be noted:

- *Loss of consciousness.* This applies, of course, only if the patient was not already unconscious.

- *Cessation of respiration.* If action is not taken quickly enough following cardiac arrest, then respiratory arrest will follow.

Treatment of cardiac arrest. If these signs are present, **immediate action** is required. The techniques of cardiopulmonary resuscitation are described in Chapter 11.

Gastrointestinal complications

Some anaesthetic agents predispose to nausea and vomiting in the postoperative period. The problem is common after diethyl ether. Modern anaesthetic techniques cause less vomiting, but every method carries some risk.

Inhalation of gastric contents results in sudden death from drowning or acute hypoxia from laryngeal or bronchial spasm. A late result may be the development of pulmonary collapse, pneumonia or lung abscess. One group of patients, in whom inhalation of foreign material is particularly likely, deserves special mention. When the pharynx and vocal cords have been anaesthetized by topical application of an analgesic agent, for example lignocaine 4%, to facilitate endoscopy, the loss of sensation often exceeds the actual operating time by up to 2 hours. Thus fluids or solids must not be given until the analgesic has ceased to act, lest they are inhaled when the patient attempts to swallow. A simple label on the patient's forehead, indicating that a topical analgesic has been used, is a useful precaution. Under this heading it should be remembered that blood in the pharynx may be inhaled to the lung also.

Preventive measures. Wherever possible, the stomach should be empty before operation. Even when a gastric tube is left in place after operation, regurgitation may still take place alongside the tube, particularly if drainage is not free, for example if a clamp or spigot is left on the upper end of the tube.

The dangers of regurgitation may be prevented to some extent by correct posturing of the patient in the tonsillar position (Fig. 6.3).

If regurgitation does occur:

1. *Keep the head low.* This ensures that all the material will flow out of the mouth and will not enter the respiratory tract.
2. *Clear the mouth and pharynx* with swabs or suction.
3. Having cleared the airway, *ensure that breathing is adequate.* If cyanosis persists, administer oxygen.

4. If there is evidence that stomach contents have been inhaled, more active measures are indicated (see p. 129).

Renal complications

It has been said that one unnecessary risk to the critically ill patient could be avoided if as much attention was paid to measurement of urine flow as to changes in pulse rate. Normally functioning kidneys are essential not only to body water and electrolyte balance but also to acid-base homeostasis. Incipient renal failure may pass unnoticed in the immediate postoperative period unless there is a proper understanding of its mechanisms and a recognition of the conditions in which it is likely to occur.

A simple classification of renal failure is:

Prerenal—where there is severe dehydration or loss of circulatory blood volume

Intrinsic—where the renal tissue itself suffers damage which may or may not be reversible

Postrenal—for example, where bilateral calculi, tumour or some other external compression as a result of surgical operation has obstructed the ureters.

We are concerned here only with the prerenal and intrinsic types. In the prerenal type of failure, which is commonly met with in the surgical patient, treatment consists of adequate restoration of the circulating blood volume, replacement of fluids and correction of electrolyte deficiencies. This will usually result in a return of normal urine flow from the previous oliguric state. Uncorrected or undetected, the prerenal type of failure can progress to the intrinsic variety, and failure to secure a normal urine flow (*at least 30 ml and preferably 50 ml per hour in the adult*) following restoration of the circulating blood volume may indicate that intrinsic failure is already established. Even at this stage the situation may be reversible if a diuretic such as 20% mannitol is given intravenously. 100 ml may be given to a maximum of three times. Failure to respond to this therapy is an indication for further treatment by a renal physician, which may be conservative or may include haemodialysis until normal renal function returns.

The predisposing factors are:

- Reduced renal blood flow resulting from a reduction in circulating blood volume

- Metabolic acidosis, which is almost invariably present in the shocked patient
- Excessive circulating haemoglobin or myoglobin as is commonly found in grave multiple injuries or following transfusion of incompatible blood
- Sepsis
- Surgery on the aorta at or above the level of the renal vessels.

Close observation of patients at risk is essential in the immediate postoperative phase and should consist of hourly urine volume measurement along with blood pressure and central venous pressure measurements. Frequent measurements to detect any metabolic acidosis are important, as is the measurement of urine and plasma osmolality. The ratio of urine to plasma osmolality taken in conjunction with hourly urine flow is valuable in the detection of early acute reversible intrinsic renal failure and its differentiation from prerenal failure. A ratio of more than 2 : 1 denotes prerenal failure, while a ratio progressively less than 1.7 : 1 indicates early to established intrinsic renal failure.

Neurological sequelae

Although neurological complications of anaesthesia are relatively rare, many are preventable if due care and attention are paid to the preparation of the patient for anaesthesia and intraoperative management. The following are some examples of this type of complication:

— *Cerebral damage* due to prolonged hypotension or other causes of cerebral hypoxia.
— *Drug-induced damage*. Lower motor neurone lesions may occur in patients with unrecognized porphyria who have been given drugs which trigger porphyria, such as barbiturates.
— *Direct damage to nerve tissue*. This can follow injection to the spinal canal where the cauda equina is injured by the needle. The median nerve may be damaged at the antecubital fossa if an intravenous injection or an irritant drug such as sodium thiopentone is misplaced. Cranial and peripheral nerves can be damaged if care is not taken with the positioning of a patient on the operating table or if the anaesthetic tubing, etc., is not adequately padded. Examples include supraorbital nerve damage by apparatus, and lateral popliteal and brachial plexus damage from the use of operating table supports.

Corneal abrasions can occur as a result of accidental trauma when the eyes are open during anaesthesia; as a safeguard against this it is good practice to tape the eyelids closed during the operation.

CARE OF SPECIAL CASES IN THE RECOVERY ROOM

Extradural and subarachnoid analgesia

These analgesic techniques interfere with three important functions of the patient's normal defence mechanism, and this state of affairs often persists well into the recovery period.

Analgesia. The regions of the body, and particularly the skin, served by the nerves which have been blocked as they leave the subarachnoid (spinal) or extradural spaces, may still be partially or completely affected after operation. As cutaneous sensation is impaired the patient will not respond normally to pain, heat or cold. Thus contact with a rough projection on the bed or a heated surface could result in traumatic ulceration or burns.

Reflexes. The normal postural reflexes will be depressed. These reflexes normally prevent overstretching of muscles or over-extension of joints. Damage can result if the limbs are allowed to remain in abnormal positions for long periods.

The use of ripple mattresses is of great assistance in the prevention of bed sores in any patient where the one posture is, of necessity, maintained for a long time. An alternative to the ripple mattress is the medical sheepskin which supports the patient on a cushion of air trapped among the fibres of the material.

Sympathetic blockade. Under sympathetic blockade the normal control of the peripheral blood vessels, which helps to maintain the blood pressure at the normal levels, is temporarily lost. Thus, blood pools in the dependent parts of the body and a severe fall in blood pressure occur. Therefore, patients under the influence of a spinal or epidural analgesic must be nursed in the recumbent position and occasionally in the head-down position until the normal tone returns to the cardiovascular system.

There are other points to observe in the management of such cases:

Headache. This is a troublesome complication following subarachnoid block, and its cause is obscure. The headache is severe, is aggravated by rising from the supine position, and may last for several days. It is commoner in younger patients and when a relatively large-bore needle has been used. There are several recommendations for the treatment of spinal headache, as the condition is called. At present the most widely used is the injection of a small quantity of the patient's own blood to the extradural space near to the point of previous injection. It is generally considered that this forms a seal of the previously perforated dura-arachnoid. In many cases the recovery from headache is impressively rapid.

Acute retention of urine. This can occur particularly in older men with prostatic enlargement. However, while the analgesic effect persists, the distended bladder does not cause undue discomfort. The abdomen therefore should be examined regularly for any sign of bladder distension, and catheterization may be required.

Sterility. Particular care must be taken of patients in whom continuous extradural analgesia is maintained after operation. Those responsible for the maintenance of syringes and for giving injections should ensure absolute sterility. The syringe should be filled under sterile conditions, and a bacterial filter is placed between the syringe and the catheter through which the injection is given.

Induced hypotension

Some surgical procedures are facilitated if bleeding in the field of operation is reduced to a minimum by lowering the arterial pressure deliberately during anaesthesia, for example neurosurgery, microsurgery of the middle ear and some types of plastic surgery.

The loss of vasomotor tone (dilatation of the blood vessels) produced by these methods may last well into the recovery phase and, although the patient may have become fully conscious, it is still very likely that a severe fall in pressure will occur if sitting up is allowed. Frequent pulse and blood pressure recording is therefore of the greatest importance in these patients until the hypotensive effect wears off.

Endoscopy

The diagnostic procedures of laryngoscopy, bronchoscopy, oesophagoscopy and gastroscopy may be carried out under topical (local) anaesthesia or a combination of topical and general anaesthesia. If a local anaesthetic has been given there will be a loss of sensation in the mouth, oropharynx and larynx and the cough reflex may be depressed also. Two dangers must be avoided in the recovery room:

- If solids or liquids are given by mouth, they may enter the lungs.
- Hot liquid may cause burns to the anaesthetized mucosal surface.

For a period of at least 3 hours from the start of the procedure, no fluids or solids are given to these patients, even if they are fully conscious and cooperative.

Because the cough reflex may be impaired, secretions tend to accumulate in the mouth and airway and patients must be encouraged to cough them up or, if necessary, they must be removed by gentle suction. The use of the tonsillar position in bed, even when the patient is fully conscious, is recommended.

Thoracotomy

The two most dangerous complications are unrecognized bleeding inside the chest resulting in a *haemothorax*, and air inside the chest escaping from a damaged area of lung resulting in *pneumothorax*. The presence of blood or air in quantity within the pleural cavity causes collapse of the underlying lung, resulting in inadequate ventilation. Because of these dangers a drain is usually inserted by the surgeon into the pleural cavity at the end of the operation. If this were an ordinary tube drain such as is commonly used following abdominal surgery, air would be sucked into the chest during inspiration and the lung would collapse.

There are three variations of the water-sealed or closed drain in common use. The first of these is illustrated in Figure 9.3 and is the method most commonly employed. Where large quantities of blood or fluid are expected, a second collecting bottle can be interposed between the water-sealed bottle and the patient. This enables a more precise measurement of the blood loss to be made when the collecting bottle is suitably calibrated.

The third method of drainage is used in situations where it is desirable to be able to control the negative pressure within the water-sealed system in order to keep the lung fully expanded (Fig. 9.4). This time the second bottle is on the opposite side of the water-sealed bottle from the patient and has an additional tube open to the atmosphere at one end and submerged 5–10 cm below the surface of the sterile liquid at the other. Adjustment of this tube at different depths below the surface maintains the negative pressure within the whole system at -5 to -10 cm H_2O when the

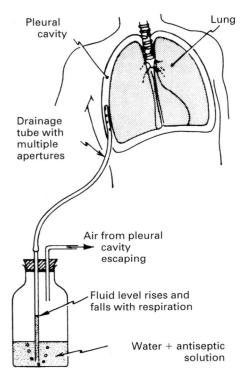

Fig. 9.3 Water-sealed drain. It is important that the chest drain be attached to the glass tube which opens under the surface of the liquid in the bottle.

bottle outlet is attached to suction apparatus and this is usually done where there is a large air-leak from the lung such as is encountered in bronchopleural fistulae. The application of a dangerously large negative pressure to the pleural cavity is avoided since if the -5 to -10 cm selected pressure is exceeded, air will be drawn into the system from the atmosphere via the open end of the third tube. When suction is used in this way, air should always be seen to be bubbling gently from the submerged end of the tube.

Although the intrathoracic catheter is generally inserted so that it lies in the lower part of the pleural cavity when blood and fluid is being drained, an apical drain is best where air is leaking from the lung. The reason for employing the higher position is that air collects in the upper pleural cavity if the patient is semi-recumbent or erect.

A word of warning is necessary. During transportation of the

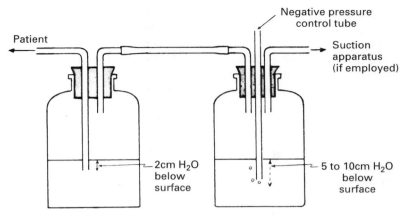

Fig. 9.4   Water-sealed system enabling the negative pressure to be adjusted as required.

patient or moving him about in bed, the bottle must always be kept at a lower level than the chest, unless the tubing is clamped, otherwise the fluid in the bottle will flow back up the tube into the chest. If the chest drain is patent, the level of the fluid in the descending glass tube will fluctuate smoothly with respiration. If it does not, then the tube is probably blocked with debris or clotted blood and must be gently 'milked' until patent again. Alternatively, a one-way valve may be attached to the chest drain (Fig. 9.5).

In this section we have described the methods of chest drainage which have been traditional and which are still used in a number of centres. These allow the student a better understanding of the basic principles. As an alternative to the use of glass bottles, there are disposable drainage collection systems which allow accurate

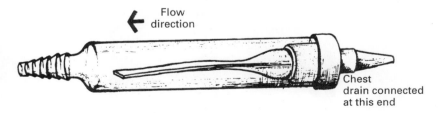

Fig. 9.5   Heimlich valve. This one-way valve is interposed between the chest drain and the drainage bottle. Air and blood may flow in the direction indicated but the rubber valve prevents air from entering the pleural cavity.

measurement of the fluid losses from the pleural space together with easy adjustment of the pressure to which the drainage tube is exposed.

Although a chest drain is usually introduced to the pleural cavity formally during open thoracotomy, there are occasions in emergency situations where a catheter has to be introduced quickly by a 'blind' technique. This is done where there has been a rapid and dangerous accumulation of air or blood in the pleural cavity, often after an injury to the chest. The catheter may be placed at the base or the apex of the cavity and this is done usually under local anaesthesia, by means of a trocar which is inserted within the catheter. Through a small skin incision the trocar and catheter are advanced between the ribs until the pleural cavity is penetrated. The trocar is then removed and the catheter connected to the water-sealed drainage bottle in the usual way. In order to facilitate positioning of the catheter it has a radiopaque strip along its length which enables it to be seen clearly on X-ray (Fig. 9.6).

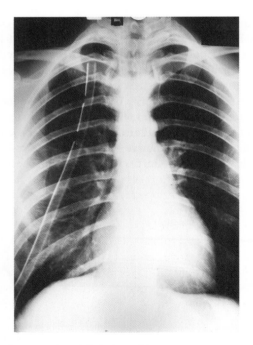

Fig. 9.6   A radiopaque pleural drain in position.

Patients who have had a thoracic operation may have considerable wound pain and pleural irritation from the chest drain. This discourages them from moving, breathing deeply or coughing. Of course, this results in retention of secretions in the bronchi and leads to hypoxia and carbon dioxide retention. Adequate doses of analgesics must be given to permit a good respiratory effort to be maintained, and coughing must be encouraged to clear the airway of secretions. Nowhere is the value of the postoperative recovery room and HDV more apparent than in the supervision of these patients.

After craniotomy

Patients who have undergone neurosurgical procedures may be conscious or unconscious. In the case of the conscious patient the problem usually resolves itself into the careful observation of the conscious level, the cardiopulmonary state and ensuring adequate nutrition. When the patient is unconscious, meticulous attention must be paid to alterations in the level of consciousness, and for this purpose a special chart is of assistance (Fig. 10.7, p. 184). Signs of increased intracranial pressure are an indication for urgent intervention to avoid irreparable cerebral damage from 'coning'. The measurement of central venous pressure is invaluable as an uncontrolled increase can result in increased intracranial pressure.

The management of the airway in those patients is of paramount importance since hypoxia or retention of carbon dioxide can increase cerebral oedema and prejudice recovery. Active cooling measures may be required where hyperthermia is a complication. Drugs used for sedation after neurosurgery or head injury may play a significant part by reducing cerebral oxygen demand when, as a result of injury or intervention, blood (and oxygen) supply is compromised.

Under some circumstances patients recovering from neurosurgery may continue to receive artificial ventilation of the lungs as part of their postoperative management. This ensures control of the arterial $P\text{CO}_2$ tension, an important determinant of intracranial pressure. It is common practice to measure the intraventricular pressure continuously in the postoperative period. This provides a very sensitive index of the intracranial state and can highlight at an early stage deleterious factors such as hypoxia, hypercarbia and the effects of haemorrhage.

OTHER POINTS IN RECOVERY ROOM MANAGEMENT

Restlessness

Restlessness during recovery from anaesthesia is common, and the diagnosis and treatment of the underlying cause may be crucial to the patient's welfare and survival. Often restlessness is interpreted as a need for sedative or analgesic drugs, but these should not be given until the cause has been determined accurately. The following are some of the possible causes of restlessness:

Inadequate ventilation. This can be diagnosed with certainty if signs of hypoxia or carbon dioxide retention are present (p. 120). Cerebral hypoxia may occur in an anaemic patient where the arterial Po_2 might be within reasonable limits but the cardiac output is unable to meet the oxygen demands of brain tissue. A similar consideration may apply in a patient who is shivering vigorously in the postoperative period since the act of shivering may increase the overall tissue oxygen demand several-fold; this problem is particularly associated with recovery from halothane anaesthesia.

Haemorrhage. A reduction in arterial pressure with tachycardia is strongly suggestive of hidden bleeding.

Pain other than wound pain. This may result from a full bladder, bladder catheters, etc.

Head injury. This may be associated with marked restlessness during the recovery phase.

Elderly patients may be restless for reasons that are not entirely obvious but which appear not to include those listed above.

When these causes have been excluded, it may be safe to assume that pain at the site of operation is responsible. In most cases, of course, the patient's verbal responses may be sufficient to indicate that this is so. Suitable analgesia should be given.

Hypothermia

During general anaesthesia the thermoregulatory mechanisms may be impaired to the point at which the body temperature begins to decrease. This is particularly likely in elderly patients and in those in whom there has been prolonged exposure of serous surfaces, such as bowel or pleura. It is good practice to be in the habit of measuring core temperature in such patients; this requires the insertion of a thermometer probe to the nasopharynx or oesophagus. Axillary and sublingual temperature measurement is a waste of time in these circumstances. Postoperative core temperatures of

34°C or even less are not uncommon after major surgery. The *prevention* of hypothermia includes the protection of serous surfaces from cooling, such as can be achieved by enclosing a major portion of the bowel in a polythene bag, the use of a heated mattress on the operating table, the warming of infusion fluids and ensuring that the temperature of the operating theatre is in the range 21–24°C. Hypothermia is a problem only if it is a factor in delaying recovery of consciousness or if it causes the patient to shiver. If the patient is wrapped in a metallized 'space' blanket, body temperature will return to the normal value in the first few hours of the recovery period.

Anxiety

This is common in patients in hospital and should not be ignored. Preoperative anxiety is one of the reasons for the use of premedicant drugs, but anxiety may occur in the postoperative period, often for good reasons, particularly in patients who have been found to have cancer or who may fear that is so. When anxiety occurs together with postoperative pain, the anxiolytic effect of a narcotic analgesic can be expected to have a two-fold benefit. Where there is no pain, postoperative anxiety may be an indication for the administration of a sedative such as diazepam. A dose of 5 mg three times per day given by mouth would be typical.

Insomnia

Many patients who have been in the habit of taking hypnotics at home may need continuation of therapy in order to ensure that sleep occurs, even if postoperative pain is not a problem. In any case the general noise and activity of the hospital ward is not conducive to sleep and it is part of good management to offer a hypnotic to patients who appear to be in need of it. There are many drugs to choose from, but nitrazepam 5–10 mg given by mouth is considered by many to be a safe hypnotic in these circumstances.

INHALATION THERAPY

The gas most commonly utilized in inhalation therapy is oxygen, although mixtures of oxygen with carbon dioxide (in carbon monoxide poisoning) or helium (in respiratory obstruction) are used occasionally. Increasing the concentration of oxygen, even to 100%, in the inspired gas or air is of limited value if respiratory obstruction or inadequate ventilation is present. Where hypoxia is present and oxygen therapy is instituted, the person who orders this treatment must ensure that the airway is clear and ventilation is adequate — or he should seek help. Delivering 100% oxygen to an apnoeic patient without ensuring a clear airway, and assisting ventilation manually or mechanically, is futile.

Rationale of oxygen therapy

Ambient air contains approximately 21% of oxygen at a partial pressure of about 20 kPa. If a patient breathes 100% oxygen, the nitrogen in the lungs is 'washed' out and the partial pressure in the lungs is increased to 80–85 kPa. Thus the pressure gradient for diffusion of oxygen across the alveolar–capillary membrane is increased greatly, more oxygen is dissolved in the plasma, and the plasma content is increased approximately seven-fold. In practice, the only means by which such high concentrations of oxygen can be delivered is via highly sophisticated mask systems, which are not normally available in hospitals, a tracheostomy or a tracheal tube. Other mask systems leak either as a deliberate part of their design or accidentally.

In a few centres facilities are available for giving oxygen at pressures greater than one atmosphere (101 kPa). These installations enjoyed a great vogue in the 1960s for the treatment of a variety of conditions, usually involving organ ischaemia. Careful trials cast doubt on the efficacy of this method and the techniques have been largely abandoned but are still used occasionally in the treatment of gas gangrene. At 3 atmospheres absolute, the plasma content of oxygen is increased to 5.6 ml/dl of plasma which, in theory, is almost sufficient to maintain life without oxygen linked to haemoglobin.

Toxic effects of oxygen

In patients with respiratory disease depending on a 'hypoxic drive' to the respiratory centre to maintain breathing, uncontrolled oxygen administration can lead to *respiratory depression* and even *apnoea*.

Prolonged oxygen therapy results in *vasoconstriction* and in neonates leads to *retrolental fibroplasia* if concentrations greater than 40% are administered.

Pulmonary damage with oedema may follow prolonged administration of 100% oxygen.

Prolonged exposure to 100% oxygen at increased ambient pressures (2–3 atmospheres) can cause *disturbance to the central nervous system with convulsions.*

Methods of administration

Fixed performance systems are designed to ensure a precisely known inspired oxygen concentration under reasonably supervised clinical circumstances. The anaesthetic breathing systems described in Chapter 3 can achieve this but are impractical for use outside the operating room. HAFOE (high air flow oxygen enrichment) systems operate by delivering a high flow of oxygen-enriched air such that, irrespective of the patient's breathing pattern, the inspired concentration of oxygen is assured. The high flow also ensures that expired gas is completely eliminated through the ventilating port.

The best known example of an HAFOE system is the *Ventimask* which operates on the Venturi principle. The delivered oxygen concentration is stamped on the mask together with the oxygen flow rate which must be delivered to ensure appropriate mixing with room air in the inlet device (Fig. 9.7).

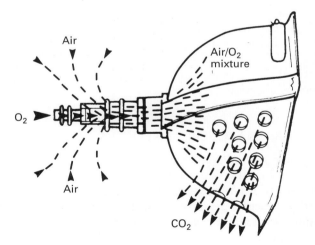

Fig. 9.7   Schematic drawing of a Ventimask. Oxygen is fed to the port marked on the left of the figure at a flow rate shown on the air entrainment device. This will ensure a fixed inspired oxygen concentration; the precise value varies according to the entrainment device used and the concentration expected is inscribed on it.

Other masks include the MC (Mary Catterall) and Hudson types. These are cheaper than the Ventimask and are often totally acceptable for postoperative oxygen therapy where the inspired oxygen concentration is not critical.

For routine correction of hypoxaemia in the postoperative period, an inspired concentration of about 35% oxygen is appropriate.

Nasal catheter. This method has the advantage of avoiding the need for a mask which may be distressing to the patient or his relatives. It has the disadvantage that the inspired oxygen concentration cannot be predicted accurately. Low flows of about 3 litre/min via a nasal catheter are well tolerated and this gives an inspired concentration of at least 25%.

In patients with chronic lung disease in whom the control of oxygen therapy may be critical, it is best to resort to occasional sampling of arterial blood for blood gas analysis to ensure both that the oxygen tension is adequate and that the arterial $P\text{CO}_2$ is not increasing progressively as a consequence of over-zealous oxygen administration.

Oxygen as a vehicle for drug administration

Bronchodilator drugs such as isoprenaline or orciprenaline can be administered in a fine droplet suspension in oxygen using a nebulizer attachment to the administration apparatus. This technique is useful in patients with bronchospasm, particularly when combined with the inhalation of mucolytic agents such as chymotrypsin or 'Alevaire' to liquefy the tenacious sputum. Antibiotics may also be administered in this way although it is more logical and efficient to give them by injection.

SEDATIVES, ANALGESICS AND HYPNOTICS

The provision of 'sedation' for patients under care is one of the first tasks to face the house officer in hospital. By definition, to sedate means to *soothe* or *settle*, but it is customary to use the term 'sedative' to describe drugs which relieve anxiety, while the terms 'analgesic' and 'hypnotic' are correctly applied to pain-relieving and sleep-producing agents respectively.

There is often an overlap in the actions of a drug; some analgesics, notably the opiates, relieving anxiety, and many sedatives, for example the benzodiazepines, in larger doses inducing sleep. It is therefore essential in selecting the appropriate drug to decide whether the aim is to remedy pain, anxiety or restlessness. It must be remembered also that if a drug is prescribed within a few hours of the beginning or end of an operation it may interact with other drugs used during anaesthesia, producing deeper or longer sleep than expected or more severe depression of blood pressure or respiration than is desirable, or both. For the safety of the patient, the house officer and the anaesthetist should cooperate in deciding what drugs are to be given immediately before and after operation.

Pain relief

If pain is present an analgesic should be administered. For milder or more chronic pain one may use tablets of codeine phosphate or paracetamol, one to two orally 4-hourly. Pain of greater severity may respond to one or other of the non-steroidal analgesics.

For severe pain, particularly in the postoperative period, the opiates or pethidine are still the drugs of choice. Morphine sulphate 10–15 mg or pethidine 50–100 mg can be given parenterally for the average adult patient (70 kg body weight). Pentazocine is claimed to be a non-addicting analgesic and is related to the opiate antagonist nalorphine. It may induce hallucinations in some patients and its duration of action is shorter than that of morphine, but the incidence of emetic sequelae is considerably less. In the UK it is now rarely used.

The combination of morphine and cyclizine (Cyclimorph) is worth considering in patients who are experiencing severe pain but who suffer nausea and vomiting when opiates are used to relieve the pain. In selecting *the correct dose* consideration should be given to the patient's physical state, his weight and any other drugs given recently. Many anaesthetists give the first postoperative dose of analgesic in dilute solution intravenously, for example morphine 10 mg, or pethidine 100 mg in 10 ml of water, taking several minutes to complete the injection and stopping the injection when pain is relieved. This technique is best employed initially under supervision. The opiates provide better psychic sedation than pethidine, and in equianalgesic doses (morphine 10 mg = pethidine 60–65 mg) there is little difference in side-effects, such as respiratory depression and nausea and vomiting. Papaveretum (no longer used in the UK) is claimed to produce less respiratory depression and nausea than morphine, but in equianalgesic dose the degree of respiratory and cardiovascular depression is similar. The

respiratory depression produced by all three drugs may be antago-
nized by the intravenous injection of naloxone 0.1–0.4 mg for an
average adult. Naloxone not only reverses the depressant effects of
narcotics but also abolishes the analgesia they produce. Narcotic-
induced respiratory depression can, however, be reversed without
interfering with analgesia by the intravenous administration of the
respiratory stimulant doxapram. This drug is not a true narcotic
antagonist but is useful in the postoperative period and is usually
administered by continuous intravenous infusion.

Never give benzodiazepine drugs to a patient suffering from
severe pain unless an analgesic is given at the same time. These
drugs may increase the sensitivity of the patient to pain and cause
marked restlessness. Remember also that after operation the
peripheral circulation may be impaired and absorption of an opiate
injected subcutaneously may be delayed. In these cases, and when
using larger or irritant injections, intravenous or intramuscular
injection is indicated.

Relief of anxiety may help to relieve pain, and the use of the benzodiazepines is of value. Bear in mind also the value of reassurance
and attention to bodily comfort — keeping the patient warm, for
example. Also of immense value is some form of distraction such
as conversation with other patients. Finally, for painful dressings,
premixed nitrous oxide and oxygen as used in labour (p. 196) may
be given. This may be used also to supplement narcotic therapy
preceding and during physiotherapy.

The problem of recognizing pain in patients in whom ventilation
of the lungs is being controlled mechanically is discussed on
page 171.

For the first few days after a major operation an opiate is usually
indicated but thereafter night sedation may take the form of a hypnotic along with codeine phosphate or paracetamol. The change
should be made from the more potent drugs as soon as practicable
to reduce the liability to addiction.

Concluding remarks

In the postoperative care of patients it is important that drugs given
to relieve symptoms are appropriate to the symptoms presenting:
analgesics should be given for the relief of pain, hypnotics for
insomnia, benzodiazepines for sedation. Although there is a wide
choice of drugs available under each of these headings, the doctor
should learn to use a small number of drugs effectively. Later in

the postoperative period it is important to remember the placebo effect. Pain relief can be obtained by 40% of patients from injections of saline and many patients sleep after taking inert tablets that are thought to be hypnotics. If drugs are to be given to patients they must be able to have a better effect than that of a mere placebo.

When dealing with restless patients it is important always to look for and deal with the cause, if possible. This may involve consulting a senior clinician.

In postoperative care it is essential to consider drugs that the patient has received recently. First, there is the question of drug interactions. Secondly, the patient may have been taking therapy in the preoperative period which it is essential to continue in the postoperative period.

A clear record of all drugs given and their dosage, route, time of administration and effect should be maintained. It is particularly important that when a patient is transferred from one part of the hospital to another, for example from recovery room to ward, the records are complete and easy to follow so that others who may have to continue treatment will be in the best position to do so.

Finally, in the administration of powerful narcotics for pain relief it is common but bad practice to prescribe that these should be given '4- or 6-hourly' as a routine. Not only may this lead to accumulation of unwanted effects but it may not be the best method of providing pain relief as regards the patient's subjective experience. In the administration of such drugs the quality of pain relief will be greatly enhanced if suitably qualified medical and nursing attendants are in a position to observe the patient carefully and to administer further drugs only when, and precisely when, these are necessary. Considerations of this type are part of the philosophy of the 24-hour postoperative care unit which is becoming increasingly popular in many parts of the world, and developing in the UK at the present time.

The management of acute pain

Treatment of pain after surgery is an essential part of the care of patients. It is morally and ethically wrong not to relieve pain when the means for doing so are available. In spite of this, for many years research studies persistently revealed that a significant proportion of patients in the postoperative period were dissatisfied with the quality of pain relief given. In 1990 a Commission of surgeons and anaesthetists produced a guideline on management of acute pain which has had a considerable impact on UK practice. The recommendations included charting the pain state in much the same way as had been done traditionally for pulse rate and temperature. Hospitals and units were encouraged to develop local pain policies reflecting the type of surgical work undertaken and the resources available for pain relief. There was also a call for the wider availability of High Dependency Units so that methods of pain relief might be administered more precisely and any complications of analgesic methods kept to a minimum through improved monitoring of respiratory and cardiovascular status in the postoperative period.

Acute pain management begins in the preoperative period when an explanation of the likely pattern of postoperative events is given to the patient with an indication of treatment that is likely to be offered. This type of 'counselling' can be shown to be highly beneficial to some patients.

Analgesic requirements

Although there are published recommendations on dose ranges for analgesics, in the case of opioids, dose requirements vary in apparently similar patients over a ten-fold range. The only sure way of coping with this problem is to tailor the doses of drugs and frequency of administration to the observed clinical end point that is required.

Patient controlled analgesia

The mainstay of postoperative analgesia remains the opioid drugs, particularly morphine. The typical postoperative prescription is for 10 mg to be given intramuscularly 3–4-hourly to a reasonably fit individual. Both the dose and frequency can be scaled down for the old, underweight or enfeebled patient.

One of the more interesting developments in postoperative analgesia has been the introduction of patient-controlled analgesia (PCA). There are many types of apparatus but the broad principle is that the patient receives a prearranged dose of opioid intravenously in response to patient demand, usually activation of a simple switch. PCA devices are in many cases computer-driven so that there is control over the frequency with which the patient can activate the demand together with built-in monitoring that allows recognition of failure of the intravenous line to operate satisfactorily, exhaustion of the reservoir for the opioid solution and a simple means of surveying the use of the analgesic since the pain control episode began. Figure 9.8 shows a relatively sophisticated system in which the controls can be pre-set and then locked with the syringe container for the opioid under the same locking device. Figure 9.9 shows a much simpler system in which the opioid is delivered from a latex reservoir that applies constant pressure to a feeder system leading to a fixed volume capacitor in the 'watch' device, the contents of which can be discharged into a vein as a result of simple digital pressure applied to the apparatus; a finite time for refilling of the capacitor is intended as a safeguard against acute accidental overdose. As might be expected, the use of patient-controlled analgesia provides, for the majority of patients, a better quality of pain relief than prearranged or occasional intramuscular injections. It is important, however, to monitor the pattern of breathing and in any case of doubt the pattern of oxygenation (with a pulse oximeter) to ensure that no unwanted respiratory complication is developing as a result of the opioid regimen. Figure 9.10 shows an idealized pharmacodynamic comparison of PCA and traditional i.m. injection of morphine.

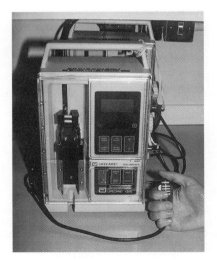

Fig. 9.8   Computer-driven apparatus for patient-controlled analgesia (PCA).

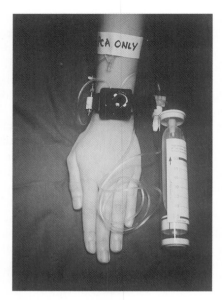

Fig. 9.9   Simple 'watch' device for PCA.

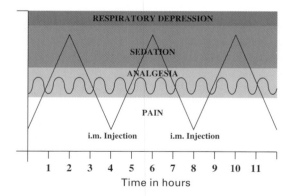

Fig. 9.10   Peaks and troughs of blood or tissue morphine concentrations (theoretical) against time in hours in the postoperative period. Note that the 'therapeutic window' of analgesia is maintained consistently with PCA (higher frequency trace); i.m. injection is either too much or too little for most of the time.

Regional analgesia

Where an indwelling catheter can be placed near to major nerves or a nerve plexus, continuous infusion of a local anaesthetic solution may provide in some cases complete pain relief through the block of all pain input. A typical example of this approach is the use of the epidural space to block lower thoracic segments after abdominal surgery. In some circumstances the combination of a dilute local anaesthetic solution with a dilute concentration of an opioid can provide high quality pain relief with the avoidance of motor nerve block which, if it occurs, can make the nursing management of the patient more difficult. The basis for giving opioids in this way is to block opioid receptors at the spinal cord level.

Inhalation analgesia

The Entonox (premixed 50% nitrous oxide in oxygen) mixture and apparatus described originally for use in obstetric analgesia (p. 196) may be useful for the control of pain in the postoperative period, particularly for acute episodes of pain such as might be associated with breathing exercises conducted by the physiotherapist, the removal of drains, etc.

Transcutaneous electrical stimulation

The administration of electrical stimuli through electrodes appropriately placed over the skin surface has brought great benefit to patients with 'chronic' pain conditions, although its use in acute pain in the postoperative period has been disappointing. From some clinics, notably in North America, there have been enthusiastic reports although the method seems difficult to reproduce in most settings. The basis of transcutaneous electrical stimulation is considered to be through the control mechanism of pain modulation at the level of the dorsal horn of the spinal cord.

Non-steroidal anti-inflammatory analgesics (NSAIDs)

NSAIDs constitute a range of compounds with anti-inflammatory activity and can be effective in many patients with postoperative pain, although their predictability in the more severe postoperative pains is less impressive than that of the opioids. There are many compounds to choose from. Ibuprofen, diclofenac and ketorolac are three examples that have been tested for the treatment of post-operative pain. The drugs can be given orally, systemically or, in some cases, rectally. A difficulty with non-steroidals is that analgesic efficacy is unpredictable. Whereas with opioids it is possible to show a crude dose response relationship for pain relief, the same is not true for NSAIDs . It is important to appreciate that NSAIDs can be associated with a wide range of toxic effects, some of which are serious or even fatal. Examples include disturbances of coagulation, gastrointestinal upset, hepatocellular and renal injury and, rarely, a troublesome and protracted bronchospasm. Although there is a risk of these complications when NSAIDs are given over a relatively short period, such as for the management of wound pain, toxicity is much more likely to be associated with protracted administration of NSAIDs, such as in the treatment of chronic arthritic conditions.

Paracetamol and paracetamol-containing compounds are not classified with NSAIDs. They may, however, be a useful addition to the armamentarium for the management of less severe or resolving postoperative pain.

Anti-emetics

Nausea and vomiting may be part of the pattern of postoperative recovery for some patients irrespective of other medication, but opioids tend to aggravate the problem. Drugs that are popular for anti-emetic use include: cyclizine hydrochloride (50 mg i.m. or i.v.), prochlorperazine (12.5 mg i.m.), metoclopramide (10 mg i.m. or i.v.). Ondansetron is a comparatively new anti-emetic which has been highly efficacious in patients undergoing certain types of cancer therapy. It is relatively expensive and few hospitals use it routinely for postoperative nausea and vomiting unless the problem persists.

Pruritus

Itching may be a troublesome problem in some patients who have received opioid analgesics and may be particularly associated with PCA and with the administration of an opioid to the spinal column. The only sure way to end the itching is to discontinue the administration of the opioid, sometimes by giving naloxone in severe cases.

If the problem is not very severe it may be worth attempting treatment with chlorpheniramine 10 mg i.m. or diluted as a slow intravenous injection.

REFERENCE

The Royal College of Surgeons of England and The College of Anaesthetists 1990 Commission on the provision of surgical services. Report of the Working Party: Pain After Surgery. September 1990

10. The intensive care unit

The concept of progressive patient care has been mentioned on page 133. An intensive care unit, sometimes referred to as intensive therapy, looks after patients who have serious illness, who need detailed and continuous observation and treatment at a level that is not available in other parts of the hospital. The patients will usually have acute failure of two or more organ systems, although some have acute respiratory failure only but require respiratory or ventilatory support for several hours or days. Originally the anaesthetist in the intensive care unit was concerned principally with the patient's respiratory problems. Nowadays the intensive care unit offers a wide range of facilities for organ support. In the UK the doctors involved in intensive care are principally drawn from the discipline of anaesthesia, but many units have a multidisciplinary team approach. The intensive care unit requires the highest standard of nursing care and of laboratory and other diagnostic support.

In this chapter we focus particularly on some of the conditions which lead to the patient's admission for respiratory intensive care. These include:

- *Postoperative respiratory insufficiency*
- *Severe head injuries and faciomaxillary injuries*
- *Trauma to the chest wall*: crushed-chest injuries
- *Chronic lung disease with respiratory failure* (chronic bronchitis or emphysema with an additional acute respiratory infection)
- *Poisoning by drugs and other chemicals*
- *Certain infectious diseases*: poliomyelitis, polyneuritis, tetanus
- *Miscellaneous medical conditions*: cerebrovascular accidents, myasthenia gravis, acute porphyria.

A proportion of patients admitted to the intensive care unit will require only general supportive therapy while under close and continuous observation. The majority, however, will require more vigorous treatment aimed at augmenting inadequate respiratory and cardiovascular function.

Mechanical assistance to ventilation (intermittent positive pressure ventilation—IPPV)

There are two main groups of patients outside of the operating theatre who require mechanical assistance to ventilation (Table 10.1):

Those with demonstrable respiratory failure. This is considered to be present if the arterial oxygen tension is less than 6.7 kPa (50 mmHg) or if the arterial carbon dioxide tension exceeds 6.7 kPa.

Those in whom respiratory failure may be confidently anticipated. Examples include patients with gross cardiopulmonary disease who are to undergo emergency surgery and extremely obese patients who are recovering from abdominal operations.

It is necessary to consider some physiological aspects of mechanical assistance to ventilation (Fig. 10.1). Controlled ventilation, whether performed manually or mechanically, has certain potentially harmful effects on the respiratory and cardiovascular systems. Excessive pressure applied to the patient's airway may result in damage to lung tissue and even rupture of the lungs. It is generally accepted that pressures exceeding 30 cmH$_2$O at the machine end of the tracheal tube or tracheostomy should be avoided, and most machines in use incorporate a safety valve or warning device which operates automatically when the airway pressure exceeds a preset value. In addition, a pressure gauge is attached to the ventilator which gives a continuous reading of the pressure at the ventilator outlet and at the attachment to the patient's airway. The volume of gases entering or leaving the lungs is monitored and displayed and may be preset by adjusting a control on the machine. Thus continuous observations of the tidal volume and cycling pressure of the ventilator and the frequency of ventilation can be made by the nurse or doctor. The patient's ventilation requirements are predicted from such factors as body weight, sex, etc., and the ventilator can be adjusted to meet these requirements. Blood gas analysis or pulse oximetry, or analysis of the expired gas in the case of carbon dioxide, can be carried out to ensure adequate oxygenation and adequate elimination of carbon dioxide.

The potentially harmful effects of IPPV on the cardiovascular system can result in a reduction in cardiac output and can lead to cardiac failure. The explanation of this is to be found when the

Table 10.1   Important causes of respiratory failure. Not all of these conditions are indications for mechanical assistance to ventilation; for example, narcotic overdose might be treated effectively with a narcotic antagonist and pneumothorax with a chest drain

Primary site affected	Causes	Examples
Central respiratory depression	Drugs	Narcotic overdose
		Self poisoning
	Hypoxia	After cardiac arrest
		Raised intracranial pressure
	Neurological disease of centre	Pickwickian syndrome (rare)
Respiratory motor neurone	Disease	Poliomyelitis
		Peripheral neuropathy
	Injury	Spinal cord compression
Neuromuscular junction	Drugs	Neuromuscular block
	Chemicals	Botulinus toxin (rare)
	Disease	Myasthenia gravis
Rib cage	Injury	Fractured ribs with flail segment
		Thoracic surgery
	Disease	Kyphoscoliosis
Diaphragm	Mechanical	Postoperative abdominal distension
		Obesity
Pleural space	Disease or injury	Pleural effusion
		Pneumothorax
		Haemothorax
Lung tissue	Disease	Chronic parenchymal disease (bronchitis and emphysema)
		Adult respiratory distress syndrome
	Injury	Lung trauma, smoke inhalation
		Inhalation of toxic fumes
	Chemicals	Acid aspiration
		Paraquat poisoning
Upper airways	Disease	Laryngeal obstruction (epiglottitis)
	Compression	Mediastinal tumours
Lower airways	Disease injury	Asthma
		Acid aspiration

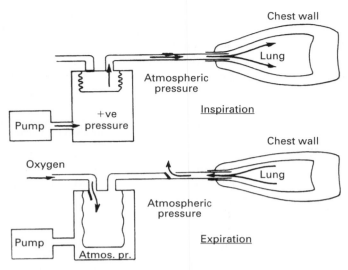

Fig. 10.1   Diagram of ventilator action: the bellows or bag containing the fresh gases are enclosed in an airtight chamber and are squeezed during inspiration by the action of a pump which raises the pressure inside the chamber above the outside or atmospheric pressure. Thus the fresh gases are propelled into the patient's lungs through the tracheal tube or tracheostomy. During expiration, the pressure in the chamber falls again to atmospheric pressure and the expired gases flow out of the lungs, escaping to the outside air through a valve. At the same time the bellows fill with fresh gas (oxygen or oxygen-enriched air) in readiness for the next inspiration.

intrathoracic pressure changes which accompany spontaneous respiration are compared with those occurring during controlled ventilation. Normally the intrapulmonary and intrapleural pressures are negative during inspiration and this assists the venous return to the right side of the heart—the 'thoracic pump' mechanism. During expiration, the intrapulmonary pressure is positive and intrapleural pressure is still negative although reduced. When controlled ventilation is undertaken, the mean intrapleural pressure is less negative and may become positive. Therefore, there is some interference with central venous return and obstruction to the pulmonary blood flow. The normal individual is able to compensate for these effects, but in severely ill or shocked patients there may be a reduction in cardiac output and hypotension.

Other patterns of mechanical ventilation can be used in selected patients. For instance, where pulmonary oedema is a problem, or where there is likely to be premature closure of the smaller bronchioles during the expiratory cycle, a positive pressure of 5–10 cmH$_2$O may be applied towards the end of this cycle of the machine. This is known as positive end-expiratory pressure (PEEP), and it must be used with great care since the effect may be to embarrass further the cardiac output. Some patients may be difficult to 'wean' from the machine following a period of ventilator therapy, and this stage in the treatment can be facilitated by arranging to augment the patient's own inadequate respiratory efforts in various ways. One method employs a 'trigger' set to change the action of the machine automatically to follow any spontaneous efforts the patient may make (patient-assisted or triggered ventilation). Another technique permits the patient to breathe spontaneously through an alternative circuit but the ventilator provides a regular boost to the patient's own breathing at a preset rate and tidal volume. This is called intermittent mandatory ventilation (IMV).

High frequency ventilation with small 'tidal' volumes may be used in some types of lung failure where circulatory embarrassment is to be minimized. The physiological basis of this type of ventilation is relatively obscure. There are three types: a frequency of one or two cycles per second; higher frequencies (high-frequency jet ventilation); and very high frequency ventilation where the air in the respiratory tract oscillates at frequencies of up to 50 cycles per second.

The manual method of ventilation, using a device such as the Ambu resuscitator (Fig. 9.2) or an anaesthetic breathing system is convenient in emergencies and for short periods of time.

The management of patients undergoing artificial ventilation

Successful management of patients undergoing artificial ventilation requires the highest standards of skill and care. Figure 10.2 summarizes some of the more important aspects.

Patients undergoing artificial ventilation will have some type of artificial airway, most commonly a tracheal tube. Although the oral route of tracheal intubation is commonly practised in the respiratory intensive care unit, there may be considerable advantages in the use of nasotracheal intubation; this allows better anchoring of the tube compared with the oral route and is thought to lessen the risk of damage to the larynx and upper trachea.

As a general rule tracheostomy is preferred to prolonged orotracheal or nasotracheal intubation. If it is thought that artificial ventilation will be required for many days and weeks, an early decision

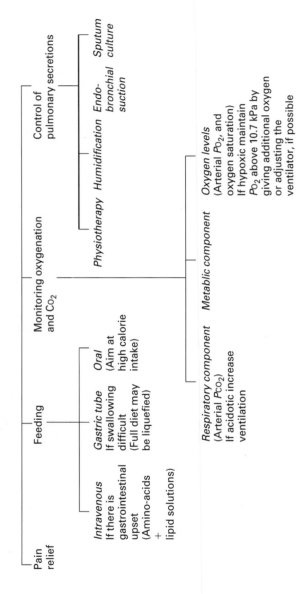

Fig. 10.2 Management of patient during artificial ventilation.

to create a tracheostomy will be taken. Often, however, the oro- or nasotracheal route is used initially and the tracheostomy created later.

The routine care of the artificial airway is of great importance, regular endobronchial suction being undertaken using sterile disposable catheters with a no-touch technique. To permit suction it is usually necessary to disconnect the lung ventilator, thus rendering the patient apnoeic, and suction should be performed in stages, allowing the patient a few breaths between each stage.

The management of pain and sedation

During ventilator therapy the provision of adequate pain relief and sedation can present difficulties, especially in the patient who is unable to communicate. Although the available drugs and techniques for pain relief are many and varied, they are of little value if the clinician is unable to detect the need for them. The patient normally reacts to unmodified pain in three ways:

- *Making avoidance movements*: attempting to withdraw the injured portion of the body from the stimulus
- *Responding autonomically*: with changes in heart rate and systolic arterial pressure and sweating
- *Responding at a cortical level* in perceiving the 'painful' stimulus and evaluating it against previous similar experience.

Many of the patients undergoing artificial ventilation are incapable of the first and third responses. Measurements of the autonomic response are as yet the only practicable approach to this difficult problem.

Remember that an immobile, apparently tranquil patient may be suffering from considerable pain and that his relief is an urgent matter. The method and drugs chosen will vary with the individual circumstances, but the possibilities are indicated below:

Parenteral analgesia and sedation. A combination of morphine and midazolam is used commonly and this may be given by continuous i.v. infusion once the needs of the patient have been determined. Infusions of propofol with an opioid are commonly used and short-acting opioids are to be preferred in some patients because they have less cumulative effect than morphine. Neuromuscular blocking drugs are very seldom used in the intensive care unit but may occasionally help in the short term if control of ventilation is difficult.

Regional blockade. Where it is possible to induce a regional block, complete analgesia of the affected part without any risk of central depression can be achieved. The treatment can be repeated at intervals or maintained continuously as in the case of extradural block.

The toxicity of prolonged exposure to nitrous oxide is a contraindication to its continuous use. Nevertheless, the Entonox mixture is of value in achieving short periods of profound analgesia for the dressing of wounds or for physiotherapy.

General care and physiotherapy

Patients must receive particular attention to pressure areas, oral hygiene, eyes and nose. The use of a ripple-mattress greatly reduces the chance of bed-sores developing. All intensive care patients have intravenous infusions which need constant attention. Passive maintenance exercises to the limbs, percussion of the chest wall and postural drainage are carried out regularly and the physiotherapist has an important role.

Tracheostomy

The indications for tracheostomy are:

— *Obstruction to the patient's upper airway.* Examples include acute oedema of the glottis and carcinoma of the larynx. Tracheostomy allows the obstruction to be by-passed and free and tranquil breathing to ensue. A tracheostomy is also fashioned in association with the operation of laryngectomy.
— *Impairment of respiratory function* in which a tracheostomy provides an artificial airway as an alternative to a nasotracheal or orotracheal tube. Tracheostomy is particularly useful as a route for the aspiration of copious secretions from the bronchial tree.

Advantages

Reduction of the physiological dead-space as a result of by-passing the upper air passage. This may have the following effects:

- Improvement of alveolar ventilation in the spontaneously breathing patient who has a limited tidal volume
- Easy removal of secretions from the air passages

- Reduction in the work of ventilation
- Better control of oxygen administration
- A ducted oxygen-enriched air supply can be connected direct to the tracheostomy tube and this can be an effective means of delivering a high inspired oxygen concentration to the patient. By contrast, mask systems are less effective in ensuring a high inspired oxygen concentration
- In patients with a depressed cough and swallowing reflex, the lungs can be *sealed off from the danger of aspirated secretions and gastric contents* by use of a cuffed tracheostomy tube (Fig. 10.3).

A tracheostomy is superior to a naso- or orotracheal tube for prolonged artificial ventilation since the tracheal tubes can cause damage to the larynx and trachea which the tracheostomy may avoid. Where a tracheostomy is likely to be necessary for a prolonged period a formal surgical dissection prior to insertion of a tube will be undertaken. In other circumstances it may be decided to use a 'percutaneous' tracheostomy using a specially designed tube with introducer which can be inserted through the cricothyroid membrane, in the midline, without the need for formal surgical dissection.

Management

Care of tubes. In the early stages a cuffed tube is preferred as it provides an effective seal for the lungs against secretions and facilitates assisted or controlled ventilation should this be required. Overinflation of the cuff for long periods can lead to excessive pressure on tracheal mucosa and to necrosis and sloughing. This can be avoided by inflation of the cuff to make a seal without excessive pressure and by deflation of the cuff at intervals for a short time. Deflation of the cuff must always be preceded by thorough oropharyngeal suction so that secretions will not run down alongside the tube into the lungs. To minimize these hazards the cuff is specially designed to ensure that high intracuff pressures cannot be achieved, so that less pressure is applied to the tracheal mucosa. It is also possible to use a double-cuffed tube, each cuff being inflated alternatively for a period. Tracheostomy tubes must be changed frequently, particularly when the sputum is copious and viscid, since the inside becomes encrusted with dried secretions. Otherwise the lumen of the tube gradually becomes blocked and the patient may die from acute asphyxia. The frequency with

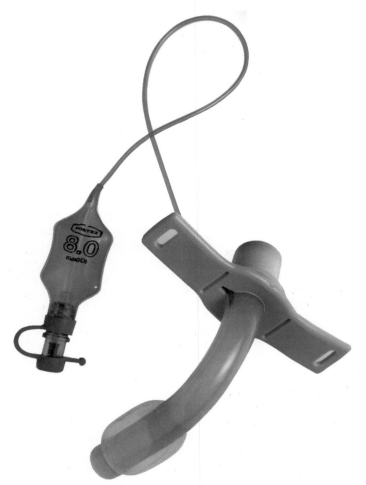

Fig. 10.3   Tracheostomy tube.

which tubes are changed varies according to the practice of the
intensive care unit, but the interval is usually 2–7 days.

Humidification. The paranasal sinuses and nasopharynx have an
important function in warming and humidifying the inspired air.
In the presence of an oral or nasotracheal tube or a tracheostomy it
is necessary to provide an alternative source of moisture and heat
to avoid hardening of the secretions and drying and fissuring of the
mucosa of the respiratory tract. This can be achieved in various
ways:

- It may be sufficient to inject small quantities (0.5 ml) of sterile saline down the tracheostomy tube at intervals.
- It may be sufficient to conserve moisture in the patient's own expired gas using a simple condenser humidifier (Fig. 10.4). The moisture in each expiration condenses on a mesh and revaporizes on inspiration. Condenser humidifiers are efficient only when the mesh remains reasonably dry and it may be necessary to change the humidifier repeatedly in the course of the day.
- In most intensive care units and in dry climates where the atmosphere contains little water vapour, or when the patient breathes oxygen-enriched air which is delivered free of moisture and fairly cold from the cylinder or pipeline, active warming and humidification are usually required.
- Other devices act like atomizers and propel a fine spray of water droplets into the stream of gas as it is inspired. These devices, known as nebulizers, operate on a variety of principles: gas driven, spinning disc or ultrasonic vibrating plate. The chief intention in the design of nebulizers is to ensure a small droplet size of 1–20 μm. An additional role of the nebulizer is to deliver various drugs in the spray such as bronchodilators (salbutamol) and antibiotics (gentamicin). In this way the drugs can be delivered into the depths of the lung.

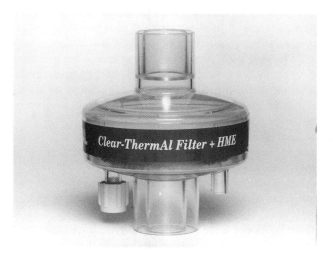

Fig. 10.4   Condenser humidifier.

Finally, humidifiers and their contents should be managed with care so as to ensure that the contents are sterile. Serious outbreaks of infection in intensive care units have been traced to contaminated humidifiers.

Endobronchial suction. The care with which secretions are aspirated from the patient's airway is of the greatest importance. The accent should always be on sterility, thoroughness and gentleness.

It is obvious that the patient is at risk from whatever lethal organism is carelessly introduced because of inadequate sterile techniques. Endobronchial catheters should be used only once and then discarded. A catheter used for oropharyngeal suction should not be used for suction through the tracheostomy. Hands should be scrupulously cleaned before each period of suction and should never come in contact with the portion of the catheter which enters the patient's airway. The doctor or nurse should wear disposable gloves.

Tracheal suction should be carried out as often as is necessary to keep the airways free from secretions. The more copious the secretions, the more often the manoeuvre must be repeated. Whenever possible, two people should cooperate during this time, one carrying out the aspiration and the other turning the patient from one side to the other to ensure that the catheter enters both right and left main bronchi.

The calibre of the catheter selected is important. Its diameter should be less than half that of the tracheostomy tube, otherwise it will block it partially or completely and cause acute asphyxia. The catheter should be occluded between finger and thumb when introduced and released to allow suction only on withdrawal, otherwise there is danger that excessive suction will collapse portions of the lung. The negative pressure should never be greater than is required to remove the secretions easily. More powerful suction is required when the sputum is thick and tenacious. At all times the catheter should be handled gently to avoid unnecessary trauma to the sensitive mucosa of the respiratory tract.

Complications

Mucosal ulceration. This occurs as a result of excessive pressure in the tracheostomy tube cuff.

Dilatation of the trachea. Overinflation of the tube cuff may result in erosion of the cartilaginous rings of the trachea and resultant dilatation.

Granuloma. Trauma to the tracheal mucosa may cause the development of granulation tissue, and a small polyp may result.

Fistula formation. This is a serious complication which may occur rarely. Excessive cuff pressure and other trauma lead to the formation of a tracheo-oesophageal fistula. Food and secretions enter the trachea below the cuff of the tube and contaminate the lungs.

Sinus formation. Imperfect healing of the post-tracheostomy stoma can result in a persistent sinus requiring surgical closure.

Erosion of blood vessels. Particularly if the stoma becomes infected, a blood vessel may be eroded by the tracheostomy tube, causing severe haemorrhage.

Tracheal stricture. In about 2% of patients with a tracheostomy and who have had ventilator treatment, a stricture may develop either at the site of the cuff or at the lower end of the tube. This is a serious late complication often requiring difficult reconstructive surgery. It is commoner in young children where the cross-section of the airway is quite small. Nasotracheal intubation is preferred to tracheostomy in children to avoid this.

Nutrition

When a patient's illness is not severe or is of short duration, inadequate nutrition may be acceptable. In patients who have suffered severe trauma and who are receiving an inadequate calorie intake, the amount of tissue protein breakdown and nitrogen loss may be two to three times that of uncomplicated starvation. For every 10 g of nitrogen excreted in the urine approximately 300 g of muscle protein is lost, and this process of catabolism is roughly proportional to the severity of surgery or trauma although the process is aggravated by the presence of sepsis. The patient in an intensive care unit who is gravely ill and in whom sepsis and abnormal electrolyte loss are present requires the most careful dietary care if a protracted stay in the unit, or indeed a fatal outcome, is to be avoided. The negative nitrogen balance which is a feature in these patients is largely reversible if nitrogen over and above the patient's normal requirement is provided.

If the patient can swallow and there is no gastrointestinal upset, conventional foodstuffs, liquidized if necessary, can be given. If the patient is unable to swallow there is a variety of special liquid preparations that can be given via a nasal gastric tube (enteral feeding). These foods should have an appropriate balance of protein, carbohydrate and fat together with a suitable balance of vitamins. Such preparations are particularly useful in patients who are recovering from a period of gastrointestinal disturbance perhaps associated with abdominal surgery. Where the patient is also suffering from a degree of renal failure, a preparation which is protein free may be used. Sometimes such preparations cause irritability of the bowel, resulting in diarrhoea. If this is not too severe, antidiarrhoeal preparations such as loperamide (Imodium) may be helpful. Nasogastric feeding of this type may be used as an alternative to parenteral feeding (see below) or as a follow-on from parenteral feeding when the patient has shown signs of bowel recovery but is still too ill to take an adequate diet by mouth.

In the management of feeding problems the services of a competent dietician may be of great value to an intensive care unit.

Parenteral feeding

When the patient cannot be fed via the alimentary tract, nutrients can be given by the intravenous route. Sometimes there may be a combination of tube feeding or oral feeding and intravenous nutrition — supplementary parenteral nutrition. Alternatively, the intravenous route may be the sole source of nutrition — total parenteral nutrition (TPN). In addition to the feeding problems which occur in the intensive care unit, TPN may be used in the preparation of severely malnourished patients who are about to undergo surgery or chemotherapy.

The general aim in TPN is to give a mixture of protein in the form of synthetic essential and non-essential amino acids to provide the building materials from which tissue proteins are constructed in the body, glucose and fat (as an emulsion) as a balanced source of energy. As an approximate guide the average adult should receive about 3000 kilocalories per day and enough amino acids to provide a nitrogen intake of about 14 g. Vitamin and trace element supplements will be needed in addition.

The constraints on parenteral nutrition include tolerance to glucose, which will require regular monitoring of the blood glucose concentration, and the administration of insulin to promote glucose utilization. Moreover, parenteral nutrition solutions are irritant to veins and must be administered to a central vein via a suitably placed long 'line' or cannula. Finally, solutions and routes for parenteral feeding should be handled with great care to ensure that they do not constitute a route of access for infection.

Table 10.2 gives one example of a parenteral feeding regimen for an average adult. Although the regimen provides some of the

Table 10.2   Example of a total parenteral feeding regimen for an average adult

Preparation	Volume (ml)	Energy (Kcal)	Contains (constituents per litre)
Vamin glucose	1500	967	Essential and non-essential amino acids Nitrogen 9.4 Electrolytes (mmol) Na^+ 50 K^+ 20 Cl^- 55
Intralipid 10%	500	550	Fractionated soya bean oil 100 g Fractionated egg phospholipid 12 g Glycerol 22.5 g
Dextrose 50%	750	1500	Dextrose 500 g
Supplements			
Addamel	10	—	Electrolytes ($Ca^2+ Mg^2+ Cl^-$) and trace elements (Fe, Zn, Mn, Cu, F, I). Added to VAMIN solution
Vitlipid	10	—	Calciferol, phytomenadione, retinol palmitate. Added to INTRALIPID emulsion.
Multibionta	10	—	Ascorbic acid, dexpanthenol nicotinamide, piridoxine HCl, riboflavine, thiamine, tocopheryl acetate, vitamin A

This regimen provides a total fluid (water) supply per day of 2780 ml. It is not adequate as a source of Na, K or Cl and these ions will be given, with additional water, according to calculated requirements.

requirements for electrolytes such as sodium and potassium, it should be realized that it is not sufficient to meet all the requirements and that supplementary administration of these ions will be needed.

Particular care is required when administering intravenous fat emulsions. Some patients may suffer an allergic reaction which will necessitate discontinuing the infusion and the administration of an antihistamine such as chlorpheniramine maleate (Piriton). Fat emulsions are also contraindicated in pregnancy, liver disease and where there is a blood disease with an increased bleeding tendency.

Parenteral feeding regimens for children are designed in accordance with the same principles as have been stated above. The child, however, with require a proportionately greater energy intake and nitrogen content than does the adult.

Recording of vital functions

In addition to the regular recording of arterial and other cardiovascular pressures, and occasionally flows, heart rate and temperature, it is important to observe closely and record certain aspects of the ventilator's performance during treatment. For each patient under treatment an ideal pattern of ventilation will have been chosen with regard to frequency, airway pressure (that is, the pressure at the patient's mouth during each respiratory cycle of the machine), the volume of gas being delivered to the patient's lungs and the respiratory mode (IPPV, IMV, PEEP, etc.). Intensive care units have a chart on which these events, together with other relevant data, are recorded. In the more advanced systems there may be automatic recording of the important variables (Figs 10.5 and 10.6). The doctor or nurse should listen with a stethoscope over both lungs, at intervals, to make sure that the gases are entering the lungs and are not being prevented from doing so by secretions in the upper airway or an obstructed tracheostomy tube.

Information about the patient's arterial blood–gas levels (Po_2, pH, Pco_2, and base excess) and oxygen saturation (Spo_2) during

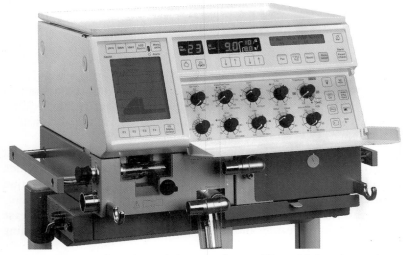

Fig. 10.5 Lung ventilator for use in intensive therapy. The sophisticated controls include delivered oxygen concentration, the inspiratory gas flow, the ratio of inspiratory to expiratory flows, and tidal volume. Monitoring displays include ventilatory profile, inspired oxygen concentration and the expired volume (V_E). Compare this ventilator with the simpler device shown in Fig. 10.6.

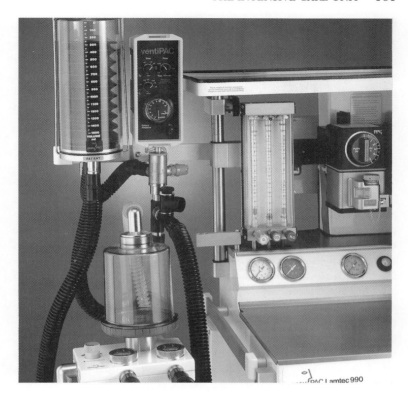

Fig. 10.6   Automatic ventilator used for patients undergoing anaesthesia. The device is integral to the anaesthetic machine. This ventilator is sometimes referred to as a 'bag-in-bottle' type. The descent of the black rubber bellows is designed to ventilate the lungs intermittently. The control box is to the right of the bellows. In the arrangement shown there is a facility for the ventilating gas to be appropriately directed into and out of the lungs via one way valves shown at the bottom of the picture. Also shown is a canister designed to contain soda lime for CO_2 absorption.

ventilation is usually recorded on the ventilation chart, and the pattern of ventilation may have to be changed at intervals to keep these levels as near to normal as possible. The maintenance of electrolyte and water balance can be difficult in such cases and it is of the utmost importance to keep *accurate* records on a suitable input–output chart. The hourly measurement of urine volume is necessary in the more severely ill, and renal function may be assessed further by regular measurement of urine and plasma osmolality.

Monitoring

In order to permit frequent, accurate measurements to be made in the most gravely ill patients, many vital functions are continuously measured and displayed electrically, or automatically charted at predetermined intervals. Alarm systems can also be incorporated to warn when heart rate or arterial pressure, etc., change beyond preset limits.

The control of infection

The operation of tracheostomy has been described as potentially lethal in that it opens up a direct route for infection to enter the patient's lungs. All open routes, such as vascular access lines, are a potential risk also. In addition, all the patients in an intensive care unit are severely ill and prone to intercurrent infection and it is therefore of the utmost importance to minimize the risk of cross-infection from one patient to the other and to isolate any cases of known severe infection by barrier nursing. Bed-stations should be at least 3–4 m apart since this measure alone greatly reduces the risk of cross-infection. To facilitate isolation of infected cases cubicles are essential, preferably with separate entrances and exits.

A further measure which is of considerable assistance is to ventilate intensive care units in the same manner as operating theatres, with filtered air from a positive pressure plenum system. Additional filters can be fitted to suction pumps and ventilator air-pumps to further safeguard the patients. All staff working in the unit should observe the accepted rules governing dress and conduct.

Modern intensive care practice depends heavily upon the support of good laboratory facilities. In the context of the control and treatment of infection, the support of an efficient bacteriological service is essential. In the management of the severely ill patient the bacteriologist may be asked to examine several specimens from a patient each day: tracheal aspirate, blood, urine, wound drainage, etc. Prompt advice on the appropriate use of antibiotics may be critical to the successful outcome of management.

The patient and the staff

Many patients undergoing artificial ventilation are fully conscious but because of a tracheostomy cannot make their wants known to the nurse or doctor in the usual way. Often they become acutely distressed and, despite continuing physical improvement, lose their will to overcome their disease. The presence of understanding and cheerful staff can go a long way towards mitigating what is, for most, a strange and terrifying experience. Some may be able to write their requests and should always have a pad of paper and pencil at hand, but for others it is necessary to provide a large alphabet on which the patient can spell out a message with a finger. Great patience is required at this stage and staff must be prepared to spend a lot of time in keeping up the patient's morale.

There are many sociological and ethical aspects to intensive care practice which are unique. The patient who is partially or fully aware during a stay in an intensive care unit may suffer a degree of psychological trauma as a result of the experience, not only in respect of illness but because of circumstances attending other patients within the intensive care unit at the same time.

The intensive care unit is a potentially terrifying and depressing place for patients' relatives who are nearly always in need of good advice, counselling and comfort as the intensive care episode progresses.

There are also psychological traumas to the nursing, medical and other staff who work in the unit. These affect different people in different ways, sometimes related to expectations for outcome that are not realized, the age of the patient (death or severe disability in a young patient is particularly poignant), and the relationship that develops with the patient and the relatives. All who work in intensive care units should be aware of how their colleagues are affected; it is an important part of good management that those who are temporarily or permanently unsuited psychologically to intensive care practice are moved to another part of the hospital.

There are many ethical issues, ranging from decisions to discontinue treatment to the prioritization of resources.

There are times when a decision is made that further active treatment is inappropriate in view of the patient's condition. In particular an instruction may be noted that in the event of circulatory arrest no attempt will be made to undertake cardiopulmonary resuscitation. When such a note is entered on a patient's record there must be a policy to review that decision at frequent intervals, probably every 24 hours. At each of these intervals the decision must be renewed or rescinded in the light of the current state of the patient's condition.

Brain death

There are occasions when there is strong reason to believe that injury or disease has resulted in brainstem death. In these circumstances, from a biological standpoint, no benefit will accrue from further artificial support because the prospect of recovery of cerebral function is non-existent. In these circumstances it is legally acceptable in Britain to declare the patient 'brain dead' and to discontinue artificial ventilation of the lungs. This is always decided in close consultation with the next of kin.

In appropriate cases in which the patient's wishes are known, or next of kin agree, organs will be removed for transplantation before life support is discontinued.

THE UNCONSCIOUS PATIENT

A varying proportion of the patients in the intensive care area are unconscious. Some may have head injuries alone while others may have additional injuries. Recording the level of unconsciousness is important and may be difficult. Accurate observations recorded frequently can be invaluable in assessing improvement or deterioration. The vitally important task of monitoring these patients can be much assisted if a standard method of recording changes is adopted. One such chart, developed at the Institute of Neurological Sciences in Glasgow, is illustrated in Figure 10.7. The nurse charts the 'best response' for eye-opening, speech and motor activity at regular

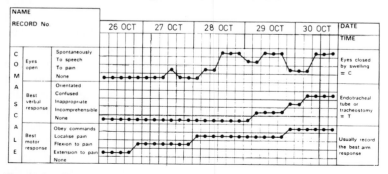

Fig. 10.7   Glasgow coma scale showing observations on a patient over a 5-day period.

intervals, and the clinician can see at a glance how the patient's neurological status is changing, if at all.

Other observations helpful in assessing these patients are rate, depth and character of respiration; rate and volume of pulse; arterial pressure and central venous pressure. In certain neurosurgical cases intracranial pressure changes can be measured directly by means of a cannula inserted through a burr-hole in the skull into the ventricle, but this, of course, carries an added risk of introducing infection.

Acute poisoning

Death from poisoning now rivals that from road accidents in the UK. About two-thirds of these deaths are non-accidental, with the number of females exceeding that of males. Accidental deaths from poisoning are almost exclusively confined to children under 10 years of age.

Of those patients who reach hospital alive, some 10% require the full facilities of an intensive care unit if they are to survive. Current patterns in acute self-poisoning show a high prevalence of benzodiazepine ingestion, with compounds obtained illegally becoming more important as a problem; many patients will have ingested more than one substance, including alcohol. Following the initial resuscitation and gastric lavage where indicated, the most important aspect of treatment is to maintain a clear airway and support respiration if this is depressed. General supportive measures may also be directed to support depressed cardiovascular function and in some patients to rewarm from a hypothermic state. The techniques already described are therefore applicable in these gravely ill patients and, if applied vigorously, are usually sufficient to ensure ultimate recovery. In certain instances, however, additional treatment is also aimed at increasing the rate of elimination of the ingested poison from the body. The availability of 24-hour poisons information services in countries such as Britain allows the doctors treating the patient to have up-to-date information on precautions and management.

11. Resuscitation: expired air resuscitation or mouth-to-mouth breathing

History

In Chapter 4 of the second Book of Kings in the Old Testament there is a description of the resuscitation of a young boy by the prophet Elisha: 'and he went up, and lay upon the child, and put his mouth upon his mouth, ... and the flesh of the child waxed warm'. For hundreds of years the method was known as Elisha breathing.

Table 11.1 shows that expired air, because of dilution by dead-space gas, has a composition closer to normal atmospheric air than does air from the lung alveoli alone. Provided that there is an adequate amount of expired air propelled into the lungs in mouth-to-mouth resuscitation, and the pulmonary blood flow is adequate, the oxygen delivery to the lung will be sufficient to ensure that the arterial haemoglobin is more than 80% saturated with oxygen; this is more than adequate to maintain the needs of the tissues for oxygen. Although expired gas contains approximately 4% carbon dioxide, an adequate ventilating volume given by mouth-to-mouth breathing will ensure effective disposal of carbon dioxide from the tissues to the atmosphere.

The process of normal ventilation can, of course, be replaced very effectively in patients with respiratory arrest using bellows such as the Ambu resuscitator to ventilate the lungs with air.

Table 11.1 Constituents of air samples (approximate values)

Gas	Atmospheric air (%)	Alveolar air (%)	Expired air (%)
Oxygen	21	14.5	14–18
Carbon dioxide	0.04	5.5	4.5
Nitrogen and water vapour	79	80	79

Provided that the operator achieves an adequate tidal volume and rate of ventilation, and the airway is clear, the arterial blood will be oxygenated to a degree that will enable tissue survival. During expired air resuscitation the donor uses his lungs and diaphragm to inflate the victim's lungs. As discussed above, the air that is delivered is not quite fresh. Nevertheless, mouth-to-mouth resuscitation is a highly effective method of maintaining life, and many patients, particularly young people, who have been the victims of accidents such as electrocution or drowning—those who have been described as having 'hearts too good to die'—have been saved because of the prompt action of someone, doctor, nurse or lay person, who was skilled in cardiopulmonary resuscitation.

The European Resuscitation Council has published basic life support guidelines on which this text is based and which should be familiar to all doctors, nurses, paramedics and public spirited lay people.

When cardiac (circulatory) arrest has occurred the patient will have collapsed unconscious with no pulse palpable (carotid, femoral, etc.) and normal breathing will have ceased. In these circumstances survival is most likely if the event is witnessed and cardiopulmonary reuscitation (CPR) is commenced immediately, if the heart arrests in ventricular fibrillation as distinct from asystole and when defibrillation is performed early. Not every collapsing or apparently unconscious patient has arrested, however. Thus, the guideline must be followed from the beginning.

In all such patients an indwelling venous cannula is essential but its insertion should not pre-empt basic CPR.

In cases of circulatory arrest, the ECG should be monitored as soon as possible.

Assessment (see also Fig. 11.3)

Gently shake the shoulders and say loudly 'Are you all right?'

If there is response or movement
Leave the person in the position in which you find him provided he is not in further danger. Check for injury. Reassess responsiveness at intervals and obtain help.

If there is no response
Shout for help.
Open the airway.

Loosen tight clothing around the neck.

Remove any obvious obstruction from the mouth, including dentures, but leave well fitting dentures in place.

Place your hand along the hairline, exerting pressure to tilt the head. Keep your thumb and index finger free to close the nose if expired air ventilation is required.

With two fingertips under the point of the chin, lift the chin; this may allow breathing to restart.

Look, listen, and feel for breathing.

Look for chest movements.

Listen for breath sounds at the mouth.

Feel for expired air at the mouth.

Wait for 5 seconds before deciding that breathing is absent.

Check for a pulse over the carotid artery in the neck. Wait for 5 seconds before deciding it is absent.

Action

Breathing present

Turn the person to the recovery position (Fig. 6.3) unless this would aggravate an injury. Check that breathing continues freely.

No breathing but pulse is present

Place person supine and give 10 breaths of expired air ventilation. Ensure that the head is tilted and chin lifted (Fig. 11.1).

Pinch the soft part of the nose closed with index finger and thumb.

Allow the mouth to open a little but maintain the chin lift.

Take a full breath and place your lips around the casualty's mouth, making sure you have a good seal.

Blow steadily into the mouth, watching for the chest to rise. Take about 2 seconds for full inflation.

Maintaining head tilt and chin lift, take your mouth away and allow the chest to fall fully as the air comes out.

Take another full breath and repeat the sequence. Give 10 such inflations in all. This should take about 1 minute.

Call for help

Return to casualty and reassess consciousness, breathing and pulse.

If a pulse is present continue ventilation alone but recheck the

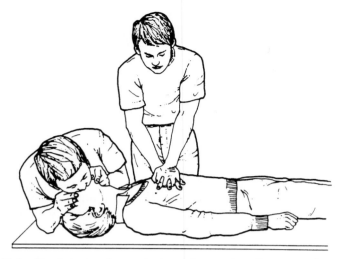

Fig. 11.1   Mouth-to-mouth resuscitation and external cardiac massage by two resuscitators in this instance. If only one person is present the position must be alternated as described in the text.

pulse after every 10 breaths, instituting cardiac resuscitation if the pulse disappears.

The tidal volume to be achieved in an adult is about 800–1200 ml, which is the amount normally required to produce visible lifting of the chest.

Only a small amount of resistance to breathing should be felt during mouth-to-mouth ventilation and each inflation should take about 2 seconds. If you try to inflate too quickly resistance will be greater, less air will get into the lungs, and gastric insufflation may occur.

Wait for the chest to fall fully during expiration before giving another inflation. This should normally take 2–4 seconds. The exact timing of expiration is not critical; wait for the chest to fall, then give another inflation. Each sequence of 10 breaths will therefore take about 40–60 seconds.

Pulse is absent

Telephone for help. The early arrival of equipment for electrical defibrillation is the victim's best chance of survival. There is no evidence that an initial precordial (chest) thump provides survival in an unwitnessed cardiac arrest. On the other hand, a witnessed or

monitored cardiac arrest may successfully be terminated by a
thump, and a thump is recommended as part of the advanced life
support protocol[1].

Place the person supine on a firm, flat surface.
Give two breaths of expired air ventilation.
Run your index and middle fingers up the lower margin of the rib
cage and locate the point where the ribs join.
With your middle finger at this point, place your index finger on
the bony sternum above.
Slide the heel of your other hand down the sternum until it
reaches your index finger. This should be the middle of the lower
half of the sternum.
Place the heel of your first hand on top of the other hand and
interlock the fingers of both hands to ensure that pressure is not
applied over the ribs (Fig. 11.2).
Lean well over the patient and, with your arms straight, press
down vertically on the sternum to depress it 4–5 cm.

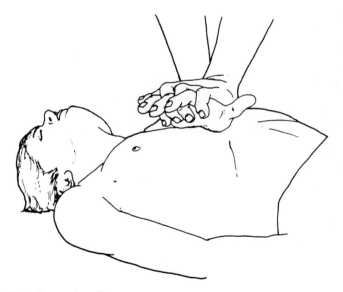

Fig. 11.2   External cardiac massage.

[1]European Resuscitation Council Working Party. Adult advanced cardiac life
support: the European Resuscitation Council guidelines 1992 (abridged) BMJ
1993; 306: 1589–93.

Release the pressure, then repeat at a rate of about 80 compressions a minute.

Combined ventilation and compression
After 15 compressions tilt the head, lift the chin and give two inflations.
Return your hands immediately to the sternum and give 15 further compressions.
Continue compressions and ventilations in a ratio of 15 : 2.

Recovery

An unconscious patient whose airway is clear and who is breathing spontaneously should be turned to the recovery position. This prevents the tongue falling back to obstruct the airway and reduces the risk of inhaling gastric contents.
Main objectives:

- Minimize movement of the patient.
- Keep the head, neck and trunk in a straight line.
- Allow gravity drainage of material from the mouth.

There is no convincing evidence that success of cardiopulmonary resuscitation is influenced by the rate of chest compressions within the range 60–100/min. Accordingly, compressions should be given at a target (mean) rate of 80/min.

As the chances are remote that effective spontaneous cardiac action will be restored by cardiopulmonary resuscitation without other techniques of advanced life support (including defibrillation),[2] time should not be wasted by further checks for a pulse. If, however, the casualty makes a movement or takes a spontaneous breath, check the carotid pulse to see whether the heart is beating;

Fig. 11.3 European Resuscitation Council's illustrated protocol for advanced cardiac life support. In particular this shows the treatment for ventricular fibrillation (VF), asystole and electromechanical dissociation (EMD). Note particularly the placement of defibrillator paddles.
(European Resuscitation Council in co-operation with Resuscitation Council (UK) © Copyright ERC 1992 Available from LAERDAL MEDICAL LTD., Laerdal House, Orpington, Kent BR6 OHX.)

---

[2]Basic Life Support Working Party of the European Resuscitation Council. Guidelines for basic life support. Resuscitation 1992; 24: 103–110.

ADVANCED CARDIAC LIFE SUPPORT

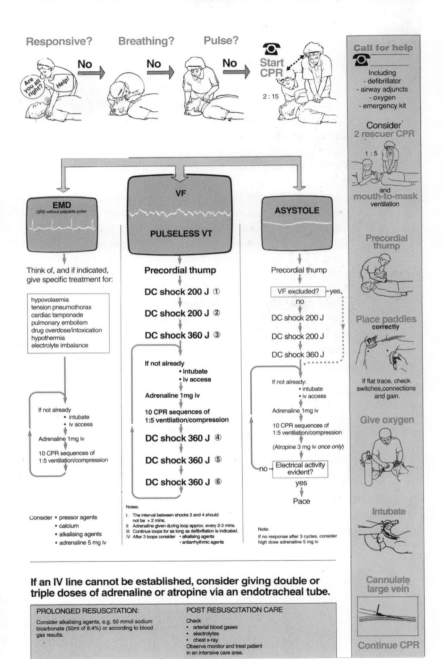

Responsive? No → **Breathing?** No → **Pulse?** No → **Start CPR** 2 : 15

Call for help
Including
- defibrillator
- airway adjuncts
- oxygen
- emergency kit

Consider 2 rescuer CPR
1 : 5
and mouth-to-mask ventilation

Precordial thump

Place paddles correctly
If flat trace, check switches, connections and gain.

Give oxygen

Intubate

Cannulate large vein

Continue CPR

EMD
QRS without palpable pulse

Think of, and if indicated, give specific treatment for:

hypovolaemia
tension pneumothorax
cardiac tamponade
pulmonary embolism
drug overdose/intoxication
hypothermia
electrolyte imbalance

If not already
- intubate
- iv access

Adrenaline 1mg iv

10 CPR sequences of 1:5 ventilation/compression

Consider • pressor agents
• calcium
• alkalising agents
• adrenaline 5 mg iv

VF / PULSELESS VT

Precordial thump

DC shock 200 J ①

DC shock 200 J ②

DC shock 360 J ③

If not already
- intubate
- iv access

Adrenaline 1mg iv

10 CPR sequences of 1:5 ventilation/compression

DC shock 360 J ④

DC shock 360 J ⑤

DC shock 360 J ⑥

Notes:
I. The interval between shocks 3 and 4 should not be > 2 mins.
II Adrenaline given during loop approx. every 2-3 mins.
III Continue loops for as long as defibrillation is indicated.
IV After 3 loops consider • alkalising agents
• antiarrhythmic agents

ASYSTOLE

Precordial thump

VF excluded? → yes
no

DC shock 200 J

DC shock 200 J

DC shock 360 J

If not already:
- intubate
- iv access

Adrenaline 1mg iv

10 CPR sequences of 1:5 ventilation/compression

(Atropine 3 mg iv once only)

Electrical activity evident?
no
yes

Pace

Note:
If no response after 3 cycles, consider high dose adrenaline 5 mg iv.

If an IV line cannot be established, consider giving double or triple doses of adrenaline or atropine via an endotracheal tube.

PROLONGED RESUSCITATION:
Consider alkalising agents, e.g. 50 mmol sodium bicarbonate (50ml of 8.4%) or according to blood gas results.

POST RESUSCITATION CARE
Check
• arterial blood gases
• electrolytes
• chest x-ray
Observe monitor and treat patient in an intensive care area.

take no more than 5 seconds. Otherwise *do not interrupt* resuscitation.

Ventricular fibrillation

This is the abnormal rhythm which is most amenable to resuscitation. It is particularly common in sudden cardiac death, for example electrocution. In addition to the basic life support described above it is now recognized that electrical defibrillation is most likely to bring a satisfactory outcome if applied early. Figure 11.3, taken from the European Resuscitation Council's guidelines, shows that in monitored venticular fibrillation or pulseless ventricular tachycardia, and with monitoring of the ECG, a precordial thump should be given. This is followed by a defibrillation sequence of two shocks at 200 joules followed by a third at 360 joules. These three shocks should be given in rapid succession, stopping only to check pulse and ECG for 5 seconds between defibrillations. There should be no return to basic life support between shocks except in the case of equipment malfunction. After three 'loops', if failure persists consideration should be given to administering sodium bicarbonate up to 50 mmol to counteract any developing acidosis, and to the use of anti-arrhythmic agents. Adrenaline 1 mg i.v. promotes vasoconstriction which will maximize blood flow to brain and myocardium.

Asystole

The algorithm shown in Fig. 11.3 applies. It should be realized that in most circumstances cardiac arrest in asystole is associated with a very much poorer outcome than following fibrillation.

It is important that all medical and paramedical personnel be fully familiar with local guidelines, know where to find all the necessary equipment, and are familiar with the safe operation of the defibrillator.

12. Anaesthetic and analgesia techniques in operative obstetrics

The administration of anaesthetics in obstetric cases has many hazards, since two separate patients — the mother and the child — have to be considered. Not infrequently, the fact that an anaesthetic is required at all for some operative procedure is also an indication that neither the mother nor the child is in the best of condition for anaesthesia. Many of the indications for caesarean section and even for forceps delivery are those involving some condition adversely affecting the fetus; for instance, antepartum haemorrhage, where the placental circulation is interfered with, or prolonged labour, where there has been undue compression of the fetus, are likely causes of hypoxia in the child. In addition, the mother may be suffering from some complication of pregnancy and may have a full or half-full stomach. The large, pregnant uterus embarrasses respiration, and the position on the table required for some procedures, for example forceps deliveries, is such that respiration is further embarrassed.

Uterine compression of the inferior vena cava may reduce cardiac output by slowing venous return. The conscious patient may feel faint and the anaesthetized patient may exhibit a marked fall in arterial pressure.

Before passing to the consideration of the anaesthetic techniques used in obstetric practice, it is desirable to give some attention to the problems of providing pain relief during normal labour.

Provision of analgesia during labour

Labour is divided into three stages: the first stage up to dilatation of the cervix, the second stage from then until the child is delivered, and the third till the placenta is delivered.

During the early stage of labour when the contractions of the uterus are felt as discomfort rather than pain, sometimes mild sedatives are used to control this. In some patients in whom anxiety is present the use of small doses of a tranquillizer such as diazepam may be tried.

The regular severe contractions, felt as definite and increasing pains, are usually controlled by the administration of a more potent analgesic drug. The one most favoured is pethidine, given in doses of 75–150 mg intramuscularly. Morphine, which is an effective analgesic and provides some degree of sedation also, has fallen from favour because of the respiratory depression which it may cause and the likelihood that this might interfere with the onset of spontaneous breathing by the baby. Diamorphine is growing in popularity. It is now believed that the degree of respiratory depression produced by pethidine is almost as great as that produced by morphine, in the equivalent dosage. Pethidine is, however, claimed to facilitate dilatation of the cervix during labour. To overcome the respiratory depression in the baby which it causes, naloxone (Narcan) may be given.

The objections to the use of narcotic analgesic agents, because they produce depression of the fetus, can be minimized by restricting their use to the early part of labour, that is before the cervix is fully dilated. From then until delivery the patient can be given nitrous oxide in 50% oxygen.

It is possible to combine nitrous oxide and oxygen premixed in one cylinder (Entonox) such that it will normally be delivered in the same proportions and supplied on demand. If the cylinder has been exposed to severe cold — and many cylinders are stored outside even in winter — the gases may separate, and when the cylinder is almost empty lower proportions of oxygen are supplied. This can be prevented by inverting the cylinders several times before use. A special demand valve is used with the cylinder. The complete Entonox unit is shown in use in Figure 12.1.

In a minority of obstetric units small concentrations of isoflurane may be given by inhalation.

The use of these volatile or gaseous analgesics from the stage of dilatation of the cervix to delivery of the child is facilitated by the previous administrations of the non-volatile agents which have been described. This is particularly valuable where nitrous oxide and oxygen is to be administered, as the residual effects of opiate or pethidine administration supplement the weak analgesic properties of these agents. The patient should have had antenatal instruction in the use of the analgesic apparatus and should be told to take deep breaths of the mixture with the onset of pain of the contraction.

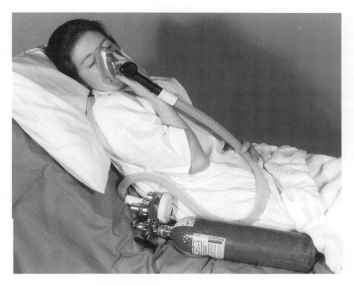

Fig. 12.1   Entonox apparatus in use.

Extradural blockade may be used to obtain pain relief during labour. This is not only valuable in relieving pain but also in allowing the cervix to dilate by encouraging maternal relaxation. In most of our major hospitals this is now the commonest method of pain relief. Nevertheless, the technique is demanding of time, and less well staffed hospitals may not be able to offer a comprehensive service. This unevenness in health care is one of the unresolved dilemmas of obstetric services at the present time.

Hypnosis and relaxation exercises

The value of relaxation during childbirth is increasingly recognized in the UK. Antenatal classes, where the patient is taught the technique of relaxation to be practised during the actual childbirth, are common. This voluntary control and relaxation of specific muscle groups is undoubtedly of value and in many patients gives considerable relief from the pains of labour. Similarly, many practitioners have found the use of hypnosis, when induced in the antenatal period and affecting the patient during labour, to be of considerable value.

At present there seems to be a revival of 'natural' methods of delivery, with some patients preferring to avoid extradural block when offered, and others gaining satisfaction and success with the 'birthing stool' which, by securing a more natural position, facilitates the birth and may reduce the severity and extent of pain. Other methods of pain relief which are currently fashionable include the (controversial) birthing pool, aromatherapy and transcutaneous electrical stimulation.

ANAESTHETIC AND ANALGESIC TECHNIQUES IN OPERATIVE OBSTETRICS

We may summarize the problems presented by the obstetric patient as follows:

- The stomach is frequently full unless there has been careful preparation to ensure a restriction of oral intake. The great fear is the risk of regurgitation and aspiration of gastric contents. As many as 10% of pregnant women may present with a hiatus hernia. This diminishes the competence of the cardia (valve mechanism at the lower end of the oesophagus), thus facilitating regurgitation.
- The position adopted for delivery hampers breathing.
- Breathing is restricted by the presence of the pregnant uterus.
- Analgesics depress the fetus.
- Obstetric manipulations embarrass breathing and may cause regurgitation.
- Some patients and their babies are in poor condition for anaesthesia. There are many causes, but cardiac disease with an insufficient cardiac output in the mother or placental insufficiency with poor oxygenation of the baby are leading factors.
- Operations and delivery in the supine position will place pressure and obstruction on the inferior vena cava leading to a reduced venous return to the right heart and a reduced cardiac output.
- *The vena caval compression syndrome.* Lateral tilt with a rubber or foam wedge under the right flank is routinely used to minimize the risk of vena caval obstruction.
- There are a number of conditions in which blood loss associated with operative obstetrics may become massive and even fatal. Effective local protocols for dealing with massive blood loss should be in place.

There are many ways of overcoming these problems during operative obstetrics. The first is to employ, where possible, some form of *local analgesia.*

Infiltration analgesia is suitable for the performance of an episiotomy or for suturing the perineum after delivery. Attention must be paid to the dose employed, as the perineum at this stage is very vascular and absorption of the local analgesic from the area may be very rapid. Only dilute solutions of the chosen analgesic are required.

Pudendal block, described on page 224, is suitable for a low forceps delivery. It is a technique which should be mastered by anyone carrying out single-handed obstetrics, as it is probably the safest technique for use in these circumstances, although it may be rather more uncomfortable for the patient than the use of a general anaesthetic. It is perhaps significant that pudendal block is the anaesthetic of choice in many obstetric hospitals.

Extradural (epidural) analgesia

This method may have been used during the earlier stages of labour, and with a catheter in the epidural space it is possible to extend its use for operative procedures. If epidural blockade has not been used before it may be instituted at this stage using the techniques described on pages 224–228. It has largely replaced paracervical block for forceps delivery because of the adverse effects the latter technique may have on the fetus. Extradural analgesia is especially valuable in cases of cervical dystocia.

Subarachnoid block (spinal analgesia)

This form of analgesia has been widely used for years, particularly for low forceps deliveries and for caesarean section. The use of subarachnoid analgesia may be associated with a fall in blood pressure which may be harmful and, if the injection spreads too far headwards, the action of the intercostal muscles may be impaired. This is particularly dangerous where the diaphragm is splinted by the large uterus and respiratory embarrassment has been noted. This has been cited as a cause of death during the performance of caesarean section under spinal analgesia. In recent years both spinal and extradural anaesthesia (analgesia) have become more popular for caesarean section in well-staffed hospitals. Much has been written about their superiority over general anaesthesia in respect of the welfare of the baby, including the importance of the mother being aware of the birth of the child as a factor in 'bonding' between mother and baby.

General anaesthesia

In most hospitals general anaesthesia is used less frequently for operative obstetrics than in the past. The hazards associated with induction of anaesthesia in the presence of a full stomach are those which have been noted previously. Routine oral antacid therapy during labour will do much to keep the stomach contents alkaline, thus avoiding the hazards of the acid aspiration syndrome (p. 129). Sodium citrate, 20 ml of 3M solution, is recommended immediately before anaesthesia or on a preoperative 2-hourly regimen if time allows. Oral H_2 blockers can also be given. Cimetidine 300 mg or ranitidine 150–300 mg may be given as early as possible before induction of anaesthesia is anticipated. The use of opioid drugs for analgesia will delay gastric emptying as may the process of labour itself. Antacid precautions should be taken before caesarean section irrespective of the method of anaesthesia intended, either general or regional.

The bed or the theatre table must be capable of tilting in any direction, so that either a head-up or head-down position can be adopted if necessary. It need hardly be stressed that, as in outpatient anaesthesia, all the normal apparatus to be found in the general operating theatre should be present in the obstetric department, namely an efficient suction apparatus, bronchoscope, fibreoptic endoscopes, anaesthetic machine and a full range of drugs and tracheal tubes.

The choice of agents used for obstetric anaesthesia varies from centre to centre but, at present, a combination very widely used is thiopentone, suxamethonium, nitrous oxide and oxygen. Premedication is usually with atropine or hyoscine only, to avoid fetal depression. In some centres diazepam is given to avoid awareness during anaesthesia. After preoxygenation, anaesthesia is induced with a small dose of thiopentone (up to 250 mg) and suxamethonium 50 mg injected intravenously. A cuffed tracheal tube is passed and inflation of the lungs is carried out with nitrous oxide and at least 33% of oxygen. A longer-acting relaxant such as vecuronium is given to facilitate controlled ventilation. If required, a small concentration of a volatile anaesthetic, such as 0.5% halothane or 1% enflurane can be given, but concentrations greater than this may depress the baby profoundly and risk uterine bleeding, since the myometrium may become excessively relaxed at high concentrations. This technique is applicable to forceps deliveries, caesarean sections and other obstetric manoeuvres, the hazards of a full stomach being present in each. Where uterine relaxation is desirable, the administration of halothane for a short time may be useful.

The use of enflurane as a supplement to nitrous oxide anaesthesia minimizes the chance of awareness during caesarean section and other procedures. Previously, awareness has been recognized as a particular problem in operative obstetrics under general anaesthesia because of an excessive reliance on nitrous oxide as the sole continuing anaesthetic (see p. 92).

The death rate associated with pregnancy and operative delivery is small but each death represents a particularly horrific tragedy. For many years in the UK there has been a systematic collection and review of information relating to such deaths, published triennially as the Confidential Enquiry into Maternal Mortality. The principal anaesthetic or anaesthetic-related causes of death at the present time include severe haemorrhage, hypotension associated with accidental overdose of local anaesthetics to the spinal column or inadvertent subarachnoid injection when an epidural injection had been intended. Other causes include failure of tracheal intubation during anaesthesia, with consequent complications leading to maternal asphyxia, and amniotic fluid embolism; eclampsia is increasingly managed by a multidisciplinary approach including an expert in obstetric intensive care who is usually an anaesthetist. In spite of the comparatively successful practice of modern times, anaesthetists who work in this particular area of obstetric care are particularly mindful of the need for the highest possible standards of management of patients at all times, the need to be aware in advance of any problems that are likely to occur and the need for constant vigilance in what may be acutely changing clinical circumstances during the management of the case.

13. Day-case anaesthesia and surgery

The practice of managing surgical operations under general anaesthesia on a day-case basis has increased greatly in the last 10 years. The principal justification is improved convenience for patients. In addition it is believed that day-case surgery makes the most efficient use of hospital resources generally, particularly beds, staff, etc. It is worth noting, however, that this operational claim is not yet clearly established.

It is important that the 'rules' for day-case surgery are clearly understood by all who work within a day-case service. There are a number of useful national and international guidelines.

Good day-case practice depends on an effective system for communication between surgeon, nurse, anaesthetist, family doctor and patient. While that requirement is common to all types of surgery, in day-case work it is recommended that the structure for communication should be based on previously agreed printed forms and letters (local guidelines).

It is usual for one member of the medical team, often the surgeon, to see and assess the patient for day-case surgery at the outpatient clinic in advance (Fig. 13.1). In many hospitals outpatient surgery is confined to patients who are in ASA grades 1 and 2 only. Those who are in other ASA categories should only be considered after careful prior consultation.

The surgery to be undertaken should be of moderate duration. Within the setting of general surgery, excision of breast lumps, herniorrhaphy and treatment for varicose veins are typical procedures. The patient should have no known adverse reactions to previous anaesthetics. Some services operate an age limit of 70 years but this is by no means universal practice.

It is important that the patient should be a reasonably responsible member of the community with a relative or friend, also capable of assuming responsibility, who will accompany the

THE ROYAL INFIRMARY
OF EDINBURGH

NHS TRUST

SURGICAL DAY BED UNIT PATIENT ASSESSMENT FORM
Part 1 to be completed by patient

Name ....   Hospital No ....

Address ....   GP Name ....

....   Address ....

Date of Birth ....

Tel No ....

Can someone accompany you home after surgery by car or taxi   yes ☐   no ☐
Does someone responsible stay in the same house with you   yes ☐   no ☐
Do you have a telephone   yes ☐   no ☐
Do you have easy access to a toilet   yes ☐   no ☐

How many stairs do you have to climb to your front door   ....

Have you ever had any surgical operations   yes ☐   no ☐
Please list:

Any anaesthetic/surgical problems   yes ☐   no ☐
Please give details:

Any other serious illnesses   yes ☐   no ☐
Please give details:

What medicines do you take ....
Have you any allergies   yes ☐   no ☐
Please give details:

Please tick box if you suffer from any of the following conditions

Chest pain on exercise or at night   ☐
Asthma, bronchitis or significant breathing problems   ☐
High blood pressure   ☐
Heart murmur   ☐
Fits or faints   ☐
Yellow jaundice   ☐
Indigestion or heartburn   ☐
Kidney or waterworks problems   ☐
Anaemia or other blood problems   ☐
Excessive bleeding or bruising   ☐
Arthritis   ☐
Neck problems   ☐
Weakness of muscles   ☐
Diabetes   ☐
Do you have a pacemaker   ☐

Do you smoke yes ☐ no ☐ if so now many per day ....

A   Do you drink alcohol yes☐ no☐ if yes how much per week ....

PART 2 TO BE COMPLETED BY SURGEON

Consultant ....

Diagnosis ....

Operation proposed ....   GA ☐   LA ☐

Patient suitable as day case ....   yes ☐   no ☐
Procedure suitable for day case ....   yes ☐   no ☐
Pre operative investigations required ....   yes ☐   no ☐
Please list.

Over 50 years of age or hypertension   ECG
Afro Caribbean   Sickle
On diuretic therapy   U&E
History of anaemia/menorrhagia   Hb

The following criteria are exclusions to Day Surgery

1. ASA III or IV (ie significant medical problems)   ☐
2. Gross obesity (body mass index greater than 32 calculated by the assessment nurse   ☐
3. Operation likely to exceed one hour (not absolute exclusion)   ☐
4. Type of procedure unsuitable (as defined by each specialty)   ☐
5. Hypertension (systolic >170mmHg, diastolic > 100mmHg)   ☐
6. Severe gastro-oesophageal reflux disease (lying flat or bending)   ☐
7. Diabetes requiring treatment or diet controlled with BM stix > 11mmol/1   ☐
8. History of anaesthetic complications and certain drugs such as MAOI's and Warfarin   ☐
9. History of asthma which requires regular treatment or previous admissions to hospital ☐
10. Sickle positive (sickle trait is OK)   ☐
11. Cervical spine or mandible problems   ☐
12. Lives outside 10 miles of RIE and does not have someone responsible to take
    them home   ☐
13. No one responsible lives in the same house   ☐
14. No or limited access to telephone   ☐
15. Poor access to toilet   ☐
16. Many stairs to climb to front door   ☐

Name of assessing doctor ....   Signature ....   Date ....

PART 3 TO BE COMPLETED BY NURSE

Patient details: Height ....   Weight ....   BMI ....   BP ....

BM stix (if diabetic ....   (if > 11mmol/1 not suitable for day surgery)

Please go through the patient's assessment in Part 1
Is the patient still suitable for day surgery   ☐
Has a date been given   ☐

What date ....   and time ....

Has the patient been given details of the operation?   ☐
Does the patient understand these?   ☐

Name of nurse ....   Signature ....   Date ....

Fig. 13.1   Example of a single sheet (two-sided) assessment form for day-case surgery.
Part 1 is completed by the patient, Part 2 by the surgeon or anaesthetist; this section is
designed to act as a trigger for four preoperative investigations: ECG, sickle cell disease or
trait (Sickledex test), estimation of urea and electrolyte content of plasma and the
haemoglobin concentration. Note the exclusion criteria listed. Part 3 is a checklist for the
nurse in charge of patient care.

patient home and be prepared to be a contact person (preferably residing with the patient) in the first 24 hours after operation. At all times the patient should understand the processes that are to be undertaken. Some services set a radius limit for the patient's home in relation to hospital: 30 miles is common. It is also important to ensure that the facilities available at home are satisfactory for a patient who may be less mobile than usual during the first 24 hours or so of recovery. For example, sleeping and toilet facilities should not involve negotiating several flights of stairs.

The best day-case facilities occur in custom-built units which admit patients for surgery early in the day and usually plan to close by 1600 h. The patient should not eat or drink on the morning of operation. It is important that most operations take place in the morning so that the patient has the benefit of the remaining day-time hours to recover and return to and settle in at home. It is bad practice to mix day-case surgery with inpatient elective surgery.

The drugs appropriate to day-case anaesthesia are those which have a short duration of action and a minimal hangover effect. Propofol is the preferred drug for i.v. induction. Nitrous oxide, any of the commonly used inhalational anaesthetics and short-acting opioids such as alfentanil are all appropriate when indicated. Day-case surgery may be facilitated by the use of local anaesthetic nerve blocks. Ilio-inguinal block is useful in herniorrhaphy, caudal block in haemorrhoidectomy. Some procedures can be carried out under local or regional analgesia alone. Alternatively, local anaesthetics may be used to lessen the likelihood of postoperative pain from the surgical incision.

In many surgical services there is a reluctance to use opioids for the management of pain after day-case surgery because such medication might limit the quality of recovery and ease of mobility for the patient preparing to go home. In particular the risk of postoperative nausea and vomiting is increased. The use of non-steroidal analgesics for postoperative pain management in the day-case patient has been a great benefit. Patients are able to take these compounds orally if appropriate. The use of non-steroidal suppositories of diclofenac allows acceptable blood levels of the drug for up to 12 hours in the postoperative period. However, there is concern that some patients have complained about the use of suppositories for postoperative pain relief without their prior knowledge that the insertion was to be undertaken. This re-emphasizes the importance of ensuring that patients are fully informed about procedures that are planned, particularly as regards consequences of which they will be aware.

14. Dental anaesthesia

In the UK, until recently, dental anaesthesia accounted for more general anaesthetics than all other branches of surgery. In recent years there has been a successful campaign to prevent anaesthetics being given in premises that were inadequately equipped, for example dental surgeries normally intended for other types of practice. This measure has led to an increase in the use of sedation combined with local anaesthetic nerve blocks and the centralization of the practice of general anaesthesia in hospitals and custom-built clinics.

Assessment

Many of the problems associated with anaesthetizing dental patients are those which are found in day-case practice described in the previous chapter. However, many of the patients come by appointment and can be presumed to arrive with an empty stomach. Some, a few of whom may have been extremely nervous, will have received mild sedation from their dentist, and this should be ascertained before commencing anaesthesia. The anaesthetist should always question the patient regarding the general medical history, particularly about untoward consequences of previous dental anaesthesia. It is essential also to be aware of any recent or current drug therapy. Physical examination may be desirable and it is regrettable that, in many types of dental anaesthetic practice, this may be impracticable.

Position

Most dental patients are anaesthetized in the dental chair, some in the supine position, others slightly head up. It is claimed that in the sitting-up position the patient may suffer a vaso-vagal attack with hypotension, and faint. The results of this can be minimized by lowering the back of the chair so that the patient is in a semirecumbent position. Ideally, however, the operation should be carried out in the supine position. Routine monitoring should include ECG, arterial pressure and pulse oximetry.

Anaesthesia

Before either anaesthesia or sedation is commenced an indwelling venous cannula should be placed and secured. Nitrous oxide is administered with adequate amounts of oxygen and a volatile supplement, normally halothane. A nasal mask such as that shown in Figure 14.1 may be used to induce anaesthesia. A mouth 'gag' or prop is inserted between the teeth, and a pack is inserted into the mouth posteriorly but not so far back as to obstruct the nasopharynx through which breathing takes place. The pack is essential not only to prevent dilution of the anaesthetic mixture by air but to prevent inhalation of blood and debris from the mouth during the anaesthesia. There have been a number of cases where recovery of consciousness has been very slow and mental impairment has followed dental anaesthesia, suggesting that cerebral hypoxia has occurred with consequent brain damage. This may be attributable to inadvertent obstruction of the airway, in spite of an appropriate inspired oxygen concentration. A mixture of nitrous oxide and oxygen alone for dental anaesthesia is seldom used except perhaps during extraction of a single anterior tooth in a child.

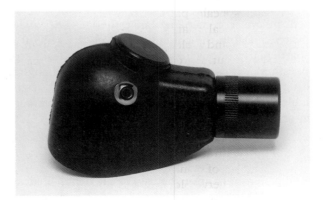

Fig. 14.1 Nasal mask.

Halothane as a supplement to nitrous oxide and oxygen anaesthesia may be maintained if necessary through a nasal mask using the nitrous oxide/oxygen–halothane mixture. However, it is standard practice in adults to induce anaesthesia with a small dose of an intravenous agent: methohexitone, etomidate or propofol. Anaesthesia is then maintained with the inhalation agents described previously. As with all outpatient procedures, adequate facilities for recovery and the return of the patient to his home must be available.

Cardiac arrhythmia during dental extractions has been demonstrated and it is considered that ventricular fibrillation or asystole may be a cause of the unexpected deaths which occur during dental anaesthesia. The value of atropine and other agents in preventing this is a matter of debate but it is generally accepted that infiltration around the base of a difficult tooth with a local analgesic is a valuable prophylactic procedure. Recent studies have suggested that the frequency of arrhythmias may be less when isoflurane is used instead of halothane; but the lesser potency of isoflurane may limit its use in this type of work in which a rapid turnover of patients is required as a rule.

ANALGESIA AND SEDATION FOR CONSERVATIVE DENTAL TREATMENT

In some patients, conservative dental procedures can be carried out more easily when the patient is sedated. To this end, some anaesthetists and dentists favour techniques whereby intermittent intravenous injections of sedatives such as diazepam or midazolam are given to produce a calm patient while the dental procedures are carried out under local analgesia. During these procedures the patient breathes air, and a clear airway must be maintained while treatment is carried out. An overdose of a sedative drug may produce a state of anaesthesia with the attendant dangers of loss of protective reflexes. The most useful guide to defining the limits of sedation are to insist that at all times the patient should be able to maintain verbal contact with the operator.

It is considered that, since any general anaesthetic carries a risk, local analgesia by infiltration or nerve block should be used where possible, and methods of combined block and sedation are encouraged widely. As with nerve blocks the practice of sedation calls for skill in handling the unexpected effects or side-effects of the drugs used: hypotension, circulatory collapse, respiratory insufficiency and bronchospasm. These problems are, happily, rare. It is important to offer a precise definition of sedation as distinct from anaesthesia: as long as the anaesthetist can maintain verbal contact with the patient, sedation can be said to exist, but loss of verbal contact is a clear sign that sedation has been excessive, that a state bordering on general anaesthesia is present and that the dangers to the patient may have increased substantially.

Major dental procedures should be undertaken under endotracheal anaesthesia in the same way as for any other operation on the head and neck. If sedation with a benzodiazepine is profound flumazenil is an effective antagonist.

A patient who is a poor anaesthetic risk for medical reasons should be admitted to hospital.

Finally, we would emphasize that practical training in dental anaesthesia is a postgraduate study to be undertaken at the hands of experts. It is our hope that such knowledge may be gained from the appropriate chapters in this book and that dental anaesthesia, while having special problems of its own, would be based on the principles that underlie good anaesthetic practice in other fields.

15. Selected local and regional techniques

Improved control of conditions for general anaesthesia and the availability of highly qualified specialist anaesthetists in the developed countries have caused a comparative decline in the use of certain well-tried methods of local and regional anaesthesia. In the last 20 years some of these methods have enjoyed a deserved return to popularity, sometimes combined with general anaesthesia. Before detailing the methods we will consider briefly their advantages and potential hazards.

A common misconception is that a local or regional technique is a completely safe alternative to general anaesthesia, for example in patients who have eaten immediately before being admitted for emergency surgery. This dangerous notion must be disposed of at the outset, since there is no guarantee that the anaesthetist will not be confronted with a toxic reaction following injection of the anaesthetic solution.

All patients presented for anaesthesia — local, regional or general — should be fully prepared in the normal manner wherever possible. Nervous patients will usually benefit from light sedation with a suitable agent. Generally speaking it is unwise to attempt these procedures in restless or drunken patients since a violent movement when a needle is introduced can have disastrous results; for example, intravascular injection to the subclavian artery or vein can occur during an attempted performance of a brachial plexus block.

The advantages of the methods are:

- The minimum of equipment is required.
- The patient can, if desired, remain conscious and cooperative.
- General anaesthesia can be avoided in patients with gross respiratory or cardiovascular disease.
- In many instances a 'dry field' can be provided for the surgeon

213

either by vasoconstriction, when adrenaline has been added to the anaesthetic solution, or in the regional techniques, by posturing the patient following the sympathetic blockade.
- Prolonged postoperative epidural analgesia can be provided by continuing the analgesia with incremental doses via an indwelling catheter.

LOCAL ANAESTHETIC AGENTS

The drugs used as local anaesthetic agents vary widely in their chemical composition; some are esters of aromatic acids, while the remainder are a miscellaneous group including amides such as lignocaine.

The mode of action of the commonly used local anaesthetics is discussed in Chapter 1. Being stored as water-soluble salts, usually the hydrochloride, with a low pH, they react with the alkaline tissues (pH 7.4) to liberate free base, thus:

$$LA : HCl + OH \rightarrow LA + Cl + H_2O$$
(free base)

The effect of this free base on the nerve is to stop conduction of impulses along it. This is the main effect and ideally the only one which should follow injection of these agents.

Side-effects and toxic effects

Side-effects are often noticeable after injection of local anaesthetic agents into the tissues or the epidural or subarachnoid spaces. It has been shown that the agent used can be detected in the blood, even in the absence of intravascular injection, and this results in a central action and the production of the unwanted effects. These are usually limited to a feeling of warmth and perhaps drowsiness due to the peripheral vasodilatation and central depression. If the patient sits or stands up he may feel faint. It should be remembered that mucosal surfaces are a highly effective route for the transmission of local anaesthetic drugs to the bloodstream; several deaths have occurred as a result of over-zealous spraying of the bronchial tree with local anaesthetic solutions in preparations for bronchoscopy.

Toxic effects may be manifest as restlessness, anxiety and confusion followed by twitchings, often proceeding to convulsions — the stage of cerebral stimulation. This may cause death by asphyxia, or may be followed by central nervous system depression with unconsciousness, respiratory depression and arterial hypotension. These effects are caused by the central action of the drug on the brain.

Sometimes, however, cardiovascular collapse may follow massive intravascular injection of the local anaesthetic. This is a result of direct action on the heart or blood vessels. Lignocaine, for example, has a well known quinidine-like action.

Treatment. At the stage of anxiety or slight twitching a small dose of diazepam may be given carefully and slowly intravenously. Oxygen should also be given. It is clearly important before the performance of any regional anaesthetic technique that an indwelling needle or cannula should be inserted into a vein.

If the patient has convulsed, diazepam or the muscle relaxant suxamethonium 50 mg should be administered intravenously and controlled ventilation with oxygen commenced. The trachea should be intubated to prevent soiling of the lungs with gastric contents. A barbiturate such as thiopentone is contraindicated when a convulsion has developed, as circulatory depression, if not already present, would follow and be aggravated by the barbiturate. Cardiovascular collapse is treated with vasopressors, plasma infusion and, if necessary, cardiac massage.

Prevention of toxic effects

Toxic effects are caused by *overdosage, intravascular injection* or *idiosyncrasy of the patient* to the normal dose of the drug.

Idiosyncrasy is rare and *intravascular injection* can be avoided by frequent attempts at aspiration through the needle.

Overdosage, the most important of the three effects, is worthy of further consideration. There is a maximum safe dose for each local anaesthetic drug beyond which toxic effects will be produced. In this respect, local anaesthetics are no different from other drugs, but failure to remember this simple fact is a frequent cause of trouble.

The safe dose varies with:

- *The drug used.* Bupivacaine is twice as potent as lignocaine.
- *The strength of solution.* The stronger solution is more rapidly absorbed and causes toxic effects more rapidly. For healthy adults (70 kg) we may use lignocaine thus:

$$60 \text{ ml of } 0.5\% = 300 \text{ mg}$$
$$25 \text{ ml of } 1.0\% = 250 \text{ mg}$$
$$10 \text{ ml of } 1.5\% = 150 \text{ mg}$$

- *The patient.* As with other drugs, reduced dosage is necessary in frail patients.
- *The site of injection.* Absorption is rapid from vascular areas, for example the perineum, and it is claimed that from inflamed mucosae absorption is almost as rapid as that following intravenous injection.
- *Adrenaline*, by delaying absorption, allows a larger dose of local analgesic to be given.

A consideration of these five factors and the extent to which they apply in any individual will be valuable in establishing the maximum dose of the local anaesthetic agent which can be given to each patient.

The drugs used

There are a large number of local anaesthetic agents available and basically they all produce their main effect — local anaesthesia — and side-effects as described in the preceding pages. Seven agents are considered in greater detail here (see also Table 15.1).

Cocaine, the first local analgesic used in clinical anaesthetic practice, is a vasoconstrictor, unlike the other agents. It is effective by injection and surface application but is extremely toxic — three times more so than lignocaine. Its use is now limited to topical application for ophthalmic and ear, nose and throat procedures in a diminishing number of hospitals.

Procaine (Novocain, Planocaine) was the most widely used drug in local analgesia in earlier times. Rapidly metabolized and only one-quarter as toxic as cocaine, it is used by injection but is not

Table 15.1 Duration of action and dosage

| Drug | Dose | | Duration of action | |
	Without adrenaline	With adrenaline	Without adrenaline	With adrenaline
Lignocaine	200 mg	500 mg	1 h	2 h
Prilocaine	400 mg	600 mg	1 h	2 h
Bupivacaine	100 mg	150 mg	5 h	No significant prolongation of action
Etidocaine	100 mg	200 mg	5 h	No significant prolongation of action

absorbed through mucous membranes except in excessive concentrations. It is therefore valueless for topical analgesia.

It has been used intravenously as an analgesic for burns dressings, to control itching and as a supplement to nitrous oxide and oxygen in patients who have received a myoneural blocking drug and who are being ventilated artificially. In addition, it has been used intravenously and intrapericardially to control cardiac arrhythmias during cardiac surgery.

Great care must be employed when giving procaine intravenously as toxic effects are easily produced. The drug is not now generally available in the UK.

Lignocaine (Xylocaine) is very stable, being little affected by heat, acids, alkalis or prolonged storage. It diffuses well, has a rapid onset of action and a more prolonged action than procaine. It is also an excellent surface analgesic. It is recommended that no more than 200 mg without, and 500 mg with, adrenaline should be given to a fit 70 kg adult. 0.25% is adequate for infiltration. Used in this way lignocaine is a safe and valuable agent.

Prilocaine (Citanest) is claimed to be 40% less toxic than lignocaine, to cause less vasodilatation and to be more rapidly metabolized. However, in addition to the other side-effects of local analgesics, with doses in excess of 600 mg (the maximum recommended dose), methaemoglobinaemia may occur. This can be treated if necessary by intravenous injection of methylene blue in equal dosage, but is a limiting factor to the more widespread use of this drug.

Bupivacaine (Marcain) is distinguished from the other local analgesic agents in common use mainly by its much greater duration of action. It would appear to be no more toxic than these other agents. In a 0.5% concentration containing 1 : 200 000 adrenaline, this drug has proved to be extremely effective for 'single-shot' extradural blockade in general surgical and obstetrical procedures, giving good analgesia for up to 5 hours.

'Heavy' Marcain is a mixture of bupivacaine hydrochloride 5 mg plus 320 mg of glucose in 4 ml. This is a hyperbaric solution; that is, it is heavier than cerebrospinal fluid. It is thus suitable for subarachnoid injection which is immediately followed by positioning of the patient to allow a degree of spread of the local anaesthetic solution under the influence of gravity.

Etidocaine (Duranest) is a long-acting drug related to lignocaine. It is stable and can be repeatedly autoclaved. The onset of action is rapid and the duration of action is similar to bupivacaine although it may be less toxic. Etidocaine may be used in concentrations of from 0.25% for local infiltration to 1.5% for extradural blockade. Concentrations as low as 0.5% produce motor blockade. Similar to bupivacaine, there is little prolongation of action by the addition of adrenaline although toxicity is probably reduced. One of the problems with etidocaine is that it may be possible to achieve motor block without complete sensory block, an unusual consequence of the use of a local anaesthetic solution.

Mepivacaine (*Carbocaine*) is in many respects similar to lignocaine although it is probably less toxic and its effect may be more prolonged. It is used for extradural block in a 1.5% solution and for subarachnoid block as a 4% solution. The maximum safe dose of the 1.5% solution is 400 mg.

Use of adrenaline

Adrenaline in dilute solution (1 : 200 000 to 1 : 400 000) is an effective vasoconstrictor when injected into the tissues. This is a valuable property when the drug is used with local anaesthetics as, with the exception of cocaine, they are all vasodilators. Vasoconstriction, by reducing the absorption of the local anaesthetic agent, prolongs its action and reduces the incidence of toxic effects with a given dose. As the local anaesthetic drugs inhibit amine oxidase, adrenaline breakdown is also retarded.

Adrenaline is, however, a dangerous substance and must be used with great care.

Locally, the vasoconstriction produced may cause ischaemic damage and systemically it may cause anxiety, restlessness, tachycardia and even ventricular fibrillation and cardiac arrest. These effects can be avoided by using the drug in 1 : 200 000 concentration, which is adequate, and by limiting the total dose for any one procedure. Stronger solutions, for example 1 : 80 000 as described in earlier editions, are unnecessary and should be avoided. Adrenaline should never be injected near to an 'end artery', for example at the base of the finger or in the ear, nose or penis.

PREPARATION FOR LOCAL OR REGIONAL ANALGESIA

No matter whether the method contemplated is local infiltration or subarachnoid analgesia, certain basic precautions should be considered.

Explanation

You should explain to the patient what you are going to do and should not subject him to a series of unexpected jabs of the needle. Failure to do so may cause unexpected pain, loss of confidence and a broken needle. In many instances the patient will, by cooperating, facilitate the location of the site of the injection.

Premedication

Before minor surgical procedures under local or regional analgesia, premedication is not usually necessary. However, in nervous patients or for major procedures a benzodiazepine is often used to allay anxiety. These drugs in the dosage employed are ineffective in preventing the twitching and convulsions seen as toxic effects of the local analgesic drugs.

The empty stomach

It is desirable that even before administering a regional anaesthetic, where consciousness is to be retained, the stomach should be empty. Where subarachnoid or epidural techniques are to be employed, coughing and clearing the pharynx may be impaired. With less extensive procedures the risk of vomiting or regurgitation must be borne in mind.

The open vein

Secure access to a convenient vein by the insertion of an indwelling cannula or the setting up of an intravenous infusion, or both, is essential. Should a toxic reaction be encountered later during the procedure, it is then possible to give appropriate intravenous medication quickly.

Checking the injection

The person giving the injection must check that the drug is the correct one, in the correct strength of solution, and that the volume to inject does not contain an overdose. Verify the presence or absence of adrenaline, noting the quantity and strength in the volume to be injected.

Asepsis

Before embarking on an injection the administrator should scrub and, except for minor infiltrations, don cap, mask, gown and gloves. The site of injection should be prepared and towelled as for a surgical operation.

SELECTED LOCAL ANALGESIC TECHNIQUES

The following are some local anaesthetic techniques in common use. The techniques of brachial plexus block and intravenous local anaesthesia are suitable for use in the accident and emergency department, while pudendal block is of great assistance to the obstetrician. Epidural analgesia is often more difficult than subarachnoid or spinal block but, unlike the other techniques described, these latter two techniques are confined to specialist anaesthetic practice.

BRACHIAL PLEXUS BLOCK

The plexus is constituted by the anterior primary divisions of C5, C6, C7, C8 and T1 with communicating branches from C4 and T2. These nerves first join into three trunks lying in the neck above the clavicle. Behind the clavicle each trunk divides into an anterior and posterior division and these unite in the axilla to form three cords (Fig. 15.1). Inferiorly, the plexus is related to the first rib, lying between the subclavian artery anteriorly and the scalenus medius behind. Anteriorly, the scalenus anterior lies in front of the upper part of the plexus and the clavicle in front of the lower part.

Technique

One of two techniques is commonly used: the supraclavicular approach or the axillary route. A third approach to the plexus, by the interscalene route, is also used by some clinicians.

The supraclavicular approach

— The patient should be sitting or lying supine with the head rotated to the opposite side and the shoulder, on the side to be blocked, depressed. This can be best accomplished if an assistant applies gentle traction to the hand and arm.

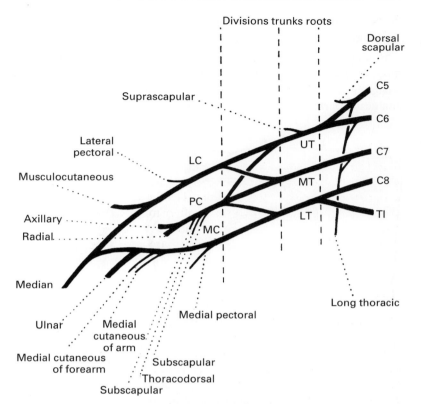

Fig. 15.1   Diagrammatic layout of the brachial plexus. UT, MT, LT: upper, middle and lower trunks; LC, PC, MC: lateral, posterior and medial cords.

— Following skin preparation with a suitable antiseptic, an intradermal wheal is raised 1 cm above the midpoint of the clavicle.
— A needle is inserted through the wheal downwards, medially and backwards until paraesthesiae are felt by the patient.
— If paraesthesiae are felt, 20–30 ml of 1% lignocaine or the equivalent dose of prilocaine is injected following a negative aspiration test.
— If paraesthesiae are not felt, then the needle is inserted until it contacts the upper surface of the first rib and 10 ml of 1% lignocaine is injected following a negative aspiration test. Three further injections of 10 ml of analgesic solution are made between the skin and the surface of the first rib,

each injection being 1 cm lateral to the preceding one (Fig. 15.2).

If the patient has experienced paraesthesiae before injection, the onset of the block is rapid, otherwise 15 minutes may elapse before analgesia is complete. Motor paralysis does not always accompany analgesia, particularly with weaker solutions.

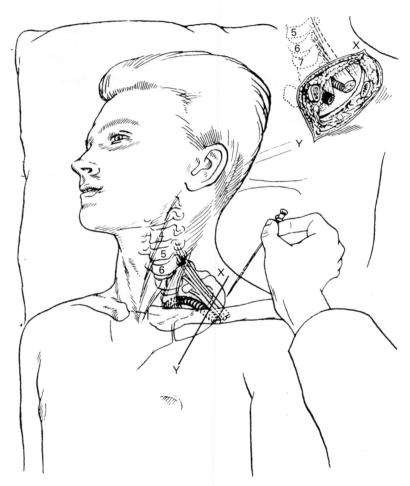

Fig. 15.2 The needle is directed backwards, medially and downwards towards the plexus lying on the first rib. *Inset:* an incision along the line XY has been made and exposes the structures crossing the first rib. The second quarter of the clavicle has been removed.

Two areas of skin are usually not anaesthetized, one on the tip of the shoulder and the other on the medial aspect of the upper arm. If surgery is contemplated on the upper arm, an additional ring of infiltration is required in this area.

The axillary approach

The main advantage of this technique is that it avoids the potential though slight risk of pneumothorax and phrenic nerve paralysis involved in the supraclavicular method. The axillary approach is also somewhat simpler:

— The patient lies supine with the arm abducted to a right angle and the elbow flexed.
— Following shaving of axillary hair and the usual skin preparation, the anaesthetist palpates the axillary artery as high in the axilla as possible.
— An intradermal wheal is raised at the selected point, proximal to the lower border of the pectoralis major muscle.
— The needle is advanced through the wheal to one side of the axillary artery, which is 'guarded' by the palpating finger, until it penetrates the axillary fascial sheath. This is usually recognized as a definite click. Following a negative aspiration test 15–20 ml of lignocaine or prilocaine 1%, with or without adrenaline 1 : 200 000, is injected. The needle is now withdrawn to the subcutaneous area and reinserted on the other side of the axillary artery where the injection is repeated, again following a negative aspiration test.

Just as in the supraclavicular technique, a subcutaneous ring of injections in the upper arm may be required if analgesia is desired on the medial aspect of the upper arm.

Brachial plexus block by either of these two routes is especially suitable for surgical procedures on the forearm and hand. If a pneumatic tourniquet is used on the upper arm, a 'dry field' can be provided which is ideal for tendon and peripheral nerve suturing.

This description of brachial plexus block serves to illustrate an important principle of nerve blocks generally — the need for an identifiable anatomical landmark. As a rule the landmark will be a bony structure, in the case of the supraclavicular block the first rib. The axillary approach to the brachial plexus illustrates how a different structure, the axillary artery, may act as an easily identifiable landmark also.

PUDENDAL NERVE BLOCK

The majority of low forceps deliveries can be accomplished if this analgesic technique is employed.

Anatomy

The pudendal nerve (S2, S3 and S4) leaves the pelvis via the greater sciatic foramen, passes across the ischial spine medial to the pudendal vessels and re-enters the pelvis via the lesser sciatic foramen. It then passes along the lateral wall of the ischiorectal fossa in a sheath of fascia (Alcock's canal). This is the region where the nerve is most accessible for infiltration with analgesic solution.

Technique

— The ischial spine is palpated vaginally with one finger.
— The fingers of the other hand are inserted into the vagina with a 20 ml syringe, containing 1% lignocaine or prilocaine with 1 : 200 000 adrenaline, held between the index and middle fingers and lying in the palm of the hand.
— The needle is inserted laterally just beyond the ischial spine to a depth of about half an inch, and following a negative aspiration test for blood,10 ml of solution is injected. The injection is repeated on the other side.

SUBARACHNOID AND EXTRADURAL ANALGESIA

It is convenient to consider the techniques of subarachnoid (spinal) analgesia and extradural analgesia together. In one method the drug is introduced into the cerebrospinal fluid in the subarachnoid space to produce motor, sensory and autonomic blockade by bathing the nerve roots as they leave the spinal cord. In the second method the local anaesthetic is introduced into the potential space immediately outside the dura mater and permeates the fatty areolar tissue there, contacting the nerves as they traverse the space (Figs 1.10 and 1.11). The actual site of action of the drug in extradural anlgesia is not known precisely but it is probable that:

• a true 'spinal' is produced by diffusion of the drug into the subarachnoid space through the dura mater, or
• the local anaesthetic acts directly on the nerve roots ensheathed in dura in the extradural space, or

• the spinal nerves are blocked in the intervertebral foramina beyond their dural sheaths.

Although extradural block is technically more difficult to perform than subarachnoid block, it may be preferred since there is a smaller chance of neurological sequelae. Spinal anaesthesia may be complicated by postoperative headache and occasional disastrous complications such as paraplegia. The latter are very rare. Nevertheless, these unpleasant results have followed apparently uneventful and meticulous procedures carried out by experts. 'Spinal headache' is much more common in younger than in older patients and when a larger-bore (22 g) needle has been used instead of a finer (26 g) needle.

SPINAL ANALGESIA OR ANAESTHESIA

Certain factors must be considered which influence the level of analgesia obtained when a drug is injected into the subarachnoid space:

The specific gravity of the solution. Cerebrospinal fluid has a specific gravity of 1001 to 1009 at body temperature, and the local anaesthetic is classified according to whether it has the same specific gravity as cerebrospinal fluid (isobaric), or a greater specific gravity (hyperbaric), or a lower specific gravity (hypobaric). Hyperbaric and hypobaric solutions will travel up or down the subarachnoid space according to whether the patient is tilted head down or head up. In practice, only hyperbaric solutions (rendered so by the addition of 5% dextrose to the preparation) and isobaric solutions are used.

The posture of the patient. As mentioned above, the posture of the patient during and for at least 15 minutes after injection will influence the level of anaesthesia obtained. The sacral and dorsal spinal curves are sites at which the solution tends to 'pool' (Fig. 15.3). If the patient is placed in the head-down position immediately after injection, there will be greater spread of the heavy solutions towards the upper segments. An extremely useful block is the so-called saddle block, performed with the patient in the sitting position; a small volume of hyperbaric solution is injected and allowed to gravitate to the sacral nerves, yielding a small area of anaesthesia particularly suited to the operation of haemorrhoidectomy.

The volume of solution injected. The height of analgesia is directly proportional to the volume of fluid injected.

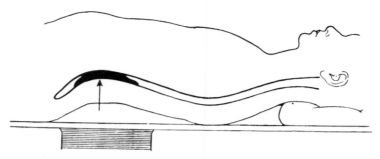

Fig. 15.3 When the patient rolls over onto his back the height of the lumbar convexity corresponds to the level L2–L3. The heavy solution now runs down both slopes. The part running into the sacral concavity is completely wasted as far as providing analgesia for abdominal surgery is concerned.

The dose of drug injected. The greater the concentration of drug, the longer will its effect last.

The force and rate of injection. A rapid and forceful injection will result in the analgesic solution travelling further along the sub-arachnoid space from the site of injection.

Some anaesthetists perform a technique known as barbotage in which in the course of the injection of a local anaesthetic solution to the cerebrospinal fluid there is intermittent withdrawal of a small quantity of the fluid, producing a type of mixing effect. Barbotage, also, is thought to extend the spread of the block.

As for most regional procedures light premedication is desirable. This allays the patient's natural anxiety and ensures a tranquil, cooperative patient during the induction of analgesia.

It is important to remember that the anaesthetic solution will not be fixed for about 15 minutes following injection, and to avoid any movement which may result in the solution travelling too high in the subarachnoid space. The progress of the anaesthesia can be determined by needle-prick of the skin of the abdominal wall, keeping in mind the segmental levels (Fig. 15.4).

Before commencing a local anaesthetic injection the anaesthetist should set up an intravenous infusion so that a ready route for drug administration is available. If a decrease in arterial pressure is not desired a suitable dose of a vasopressor such as ephedrine may be given either intramuscularly or intravenously. On the other hand the anaesthetist may be attempting to induce arterial hypotension deliberately for the purposes of minimizing blood loss or inducing a dry operative field. Many patients are content to be drowsily

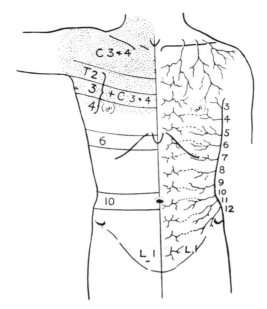

Fig. 15.4   Segmental levels of analgesia.

awake during the subsequent surgery but their eyes should be gently blindfolded. A light general anaesthetic may be administered to others and this is usually the case in upper abdominal procedures.

EXTRADURAL ANALGESIA OR ANAESTHESIA

Whereas subarachnoid injection must be made distal to the termination of the spinal cord, and the baricity of the injected solution and the posture of the patient are determinants of spread, extradural injection can be made at virtually any point in the spinal column.

The factors which influence the level of analgesia are:

The site of injection. The higher the injection the higher will be the range of segments blocked. For lower abdominal and leg procedures injection is made in the lumbar region, but for patients undergoing upper abdominal surgery and those who require pain relief after thoracic operations, and especially when prolonged analgesia is required, the injection is made in the thoracic extradural space. Here extreme care must be taken to avoid puncture of the dura-arachnoid membrane.

The rate and force of injection. Just as in subarachnoid analgesia, a rapid forceful injection will result in the solution travelling further from the site of puncture, and a higher level of analgesia will result.

The posture of the patient. A steep head-down tilt will result in the solution travelling higher and the level of analgesia will also be higher.

The volume of solution. Taller patients, having an epidural space of greater capacity, require a larger volume of solution if the same level of analgesia is to be obtained as in shorter patients.

The age of the patient. Elderly patients require a smaller volume of solution to produce any given level of analgesia.

Technique

The patient is premedicated with a sedative or an opiate as for spinal analgesia. The anaesthetist is gloved, gowned and masked and the patient's back is prepared as for any operative procedure. Two approaches are commonly used: the caudal and the lumbar.

Caudal approach (Fig. 15.5)

— The patient lies face down on the operating table or trolley with legs apart and a pillow under the pelvis. The toes should be turned inwards. This position gives the best access to the sacral hiatus.

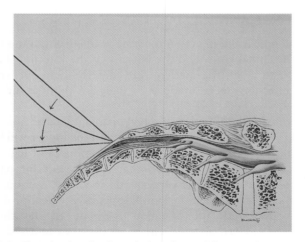

Fig. 15.5   Extradural analgesia; technique for caudal approach.

— The sacral hiatus, which results from the lack of fusion of the laminae of the fifth sacral vertebra and sometimes the fourth vertebra as well, is palpated. This is best done by sliding the finger upwards from the coccyx in the midline.

— An intradermal wheal is raised and a straight 22 gauge needle introduced at an angle of about 70–80° to the skin surface. This needle should not be more than 4.5 cm long to avoid penetration of the dural sac, which comes down to the level of the lower border of the second sacral vertebra.

— When the needle penetrates the sacrococcygeal membrane, and this is usually easy to recognize, it is depressed to an angle of 15–20° to the skin surface and it should then advance easily into the sacral canal. Two causes of failure to enter the sacral canal are:

  • The needle may be advanced superficial to the hiatus and the injection made subcutaneously with resulting swelling at the site of injection
  • The needle may be inserted under the periosteum.

— Following a negative aspiration test for cerebrospinal fluid and blood, a test dose of 5 ml of 1.5% lignocaine without adrenaline is injected.

— If no motor paralysis is evident after a period of 5 minutes, when the patient has been asked to move his toes, the rest of the injection is given. About 20 ml of 1.5% lignocaine is required for operations on the anus such as excision of a fissure or haemorrhoids. The analgesia is complete in 10 minutes and lasts for about 1 hour.

The anatomy of the caudal space is variable and the space may be loculated. This can result in unilateral analgesia.

In recent years caudal analgesia has become popular for the operation of circumcision in young children, by virtue of the prolonged postoperative analgesia which the method confers and the fact that the child may return home with its mother immediately after the operation has been completed.

Lumbar approach

To reach higher levels from the caudal approach, larger volumes of analgesic would be required with a greater risk of toxic effects. The lumbar approach is therefore preferred for abdominal procedures.

A special needle, the Tuohy needle, is used for a lumbar epidural analgesia (Fig. 15.6).

A catheter introduced through the Tuohy needle, directed up or downwards by rotation of the needle, enables continuous epidural analgesia to be administered. The catheter can be connected to a paediatric 'burette-type' intravenous set, thus ensuring absolute sterility.

This modification enables postoperative analgesia to be continued for hours or in some cases days and is a useful method in patients with severe respiratory disorders. The same technique, or the continuous caudal alternative, can be employed in labour, particularly in cases of cervical dystocia. Other therapeutic indications for continuous epidural analgesia are the relief of pain in acute pancreatitis, and the relief of pain and autonomic blockade in peripheral vascular disease and arterial embolism in the legs.

Control of arterial pressure

The autonomic blockade which follows epidural analgesia results in hypotension. This can be of great advantage to the surgeon, providing a fairly bloodless field for major procedures such as Wertheim's hysterectomy. The arterial systolic pressure must not be permitted to fall below 60 mmHg in fit patients and any blood loss must be meticulously restored. Should hypotension be contraindicated, a vasopressor such as ephedrine 15 mg can be given intramuscularly or intravenously following completion of the epidural injection.

INTRAVENOUS REGIONAL ANALGESIA

First described by Bier in 1908 this is a useful method of analgesia for emergency surgery on the limbs. For operations on the arm and hand it is preferred by many to brachial plexus block, which requires a greater degree of technical skill to accomplish and has occasional complications such as pneumothorax.

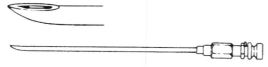

Fig. 15.6 Tuohy needle. The trocar point and side opening can be seen.

Method

A standard sphygmomanometer cuff, or a specially designed double cuff (Fig. 15.7), is placed around the patient's arm and the arterial systolic pressure recorded. A disposable plastic cannula is then introduced to a vein on the back of the hand or forearm if the hand is involved in the injury. The limb is raised and emptied of blood. This can be achieved by the application of an Esmarch bandage, working proximally from the hand to the level of the blood pressure cuff; alternatively, if the patient has a painful condition of the limb it may be sufficient simply to elevate the limb for a period to allow blood to drain from it. 40 ml (in a healthy 70 kg adult) of 0.5% prilocaine without adrenaline is then injected into the needle or cannula for an arm (i.e. lignocaine 200 mg) or up to 100 ml for a leg (i.e. 500 mg of lignocaine). Paraesthesia usually develops during the injection and is immediately followed by profound analgesia and frequently complete muscle paralysis.

On completion of the surgical procedure, power and sensation return to the limb within 5–10 minutes of release of the tourniquet.

Advantages

- It is a suitable technique for emergency procedures in patients not prepared for general anaesthesia.
- The technique is extremely simple and reliable.
- The risk of complications is much less than with brachial plexus block.

Problems can arise if the tourniquet fails immediately or soon

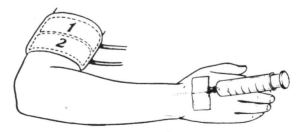

Fig. 15.7   Intravenous local analgesia. The upper cuff is inflated after the limb has been rendered bloodless. The injection is then made, the lower cuff inflated, and finally the upper one deflated.

after injection. Too rapid injection into the venous compartment may bring the intravenous pressure to a greater value than the previously measured arterial pressure, with a risk of leakage to the systemic circulation under the inflated tourniquet.

The nerves of the limb are blocked in intravenous regional analgesia by virtue of the migration of the local anaesthetic via the vascular supply to the nerve tissue itself. Once the nerve tissue has been reached a significant quantity of the injected anaesthetic is fixed for a time. Thus the tourniquet can be released after half an hour or so without a significant risk of systemic toxicity from the local anaesthetic.

16. Monitoring in anaesthesia

'Eternal vigilance is the price of safety': this is a commonly quoted free translation of the motto of the Association of Anaesthetists of Great Britain and Ireland who publish a guideline on monitoring in anaesthesia. The need for the guideline was stimulated by similar exercises in the US and in other countries, notably Australia. Various epidemiological studies had suggested an increasing number of errors in the use of anaesthetic equipment or failure to recognize important clinical signs of impending disaster during anaesthesia. Impressions were supported by some well publicized and influential medico-legal cases in the UK. These events coincided with great improvements in the design of several useful monitors and their incorporation to easy-to-use assemblies either on the anaesthetic machine itself or alongside it.

The Association of Anaesthetists' recommendations state first that the anaesthetist should be present throughout the entire period when an anaesthetic is given and should ensure that an adequate record of the procedure is made. This statement may surprise those who are unfamiliar with operating room practice but it is fair to anaesthetic specialists to emphasize that ensuring continuity of an operating list, access to drugs and other therapeutic preparations and attention to patients who are within the recovery area can all distract the anaesthetist from the safest working position: beside the patient.

The guideline further emphasizes:

- Monitoring should be commenced before induction of anaesthesia and continued until the end of recovery.
- The anaesthetic machine should have the means of allowing early recognition of failure of the oxygen supply, leaks and disconnections, or the development of high pressure within the breathing system.

- There should be continuous monitoring of the patient's ventilation and circulation.
- Appropriate monitoring should be available no matter how short the anaesthetic procedure.
- If a patient is to be transported, particularly if anaesthetized or unconscious, appropriate monitoring should be an integral part of the transport process.
- When the patient is transferred to a recovery ward or comparable area, clear instructions concerning continuing monitoring should be given and appropriate monitoring facilities should be available during recovery.

A monitoring device detects the relevant physical energy in a patient and converts (or transduces) it by means of a transducer to another energy form — usually electrical — allowing it to create a display which can be sensed by the doctor or nurse. The display may be visual or auditory, or both. Visual displays are either analogue (continuous scale, rather like a traditional watch) or digital. There may be a facility for recording the signals on paper chart, tape or disc. The same signals may be used to activate alarms if the values from the patient are outside a chosen range.

Signals may also be used to activate a therapeutic process. For example, the signal from a neuromuscular block monitor has been used experimentally to activate an electromechanical syringe so that suitable increments of a neuromuscular blocking drug are given. This is an example of *feedback control*.

The most useful monitors are those which give information on an important variable which could not be obtained by the doctor using unaided senses. We can *feel* the pulse and *observe* the pattern of breathing and, with a clock, we can count the rate of each precisely, but we cannot monitor the electric activity of the heart without an electrocardiogram (ECG).

In spite of the enormous contribution that the microelectronics industry has made to patient safety through sophisticated monitoring, it is not reactionary to say that the best monitors remain the eye, ear and finger. Instruments should complement the basic diagnostic skills, not substitute for them.

Ergonomics is the study of the effect of the working environment on performance and well-being of the worker. It is known from the aviation industry that too much information that is difficult to assimilate can, paradoxically, cause mistakes and even disasters. At present the ergonomics of monitoring, particularly warning signals, in the operating room are little understood. It is not unusual for an operating team to be subject to auditory signals that may cause confusion. These can arise from electronic paging devices, diathermy apparatus, a variety of anaesthetic monitors, and even a reversing truck outside the building.

Heart

Electrocardiography senses electric potential differences which must be amplified, associated with the excitation of cardiac muscle. Three electrodes are placed on the chest wall as far apart as possible; the precise position is unimportant. This allows detection of heart rate and rhythm. The method is not reliable for detecting subtle changes in the myocardium associated with ischaemia or infarction for which the 12-lead ECG is required.

Arterial pressures

The traditional Riva Rocci method of indirect measurement of arterial pressure remains a basic but standard method for use in many anaesthetic settings, including preoperative and postoperative assessment. Increasingly, however, automated sphygmomanometers are available, particularly in operating rooms. There are many designs, but a common arrangement involves a proximal cuff which is used to occlude and then release arterial inflow to the distal part of an arm. A distal cuff (or some other type of detector) is used to detect flow entering the distal part of the arm when the proximal cuff pressure has become less than the systolic value; with various degrees of precision these systems attempt to detect the point of decompression of the proximal cuff when pulsatile flow has reached its maximum, denoting diastolic pressure. It is relatively easy to include electronic processing which allows display of the 'mean' arterial pressure, typically diastolic pressure plus one-third of the systolic–diastolic difference.

For the more major surgical procedures a cannula is placed in an artery, usually the radial, and connected through a liquid column to a manometer or suitable transducer. Typically the resulting signal is displayed as a waveform on an oscilloscope (Fig. 16.1). Additionally, arterial pressures and derived values may be displayed digitally. It should be noted that faulty direct pressure detection systems, or faulty calibration, may lead to spurious readings. Avoid the bland assumption that once there is direct access to

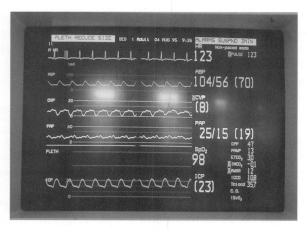

Fig. 16.1   Display of measured variables photographed from a monitor screen. From top to bottom the trace shows ECG (heart rate), arterial pressure with mean value in brackets, central venous pressure, pulmonary arterial pressure, a digital display of SpO_2, and intracranial pressure. On the bottom right of the screen are various other derived indices: $ETCO_2$ signifies that there is 3% carbon dioxide in the end tidal gas.

the arterial system the accuracy of pressure measurement is thereby improved.

Venous and other pressures

Electronic systems similar to those used for arterial pressure are used to monitor and display pressures on the venous side of the circulation. Central venous pressure measurement is sometimes a useful index of the cardiac and blood volume status. However, the interpretation of venous pressure calls for experience and careful judgement. Failure of the right ventricular pumping mechanism is likely to lead to an increase in venous pressure. Serious hypovolaemia may be associated with a decrease in venous pressure. Central venous pressure presupposes that the 'detecting' tip of the venous catheter is placed within the central veins at the level of the superior or inferior vena cava.

In some circumstances useful information can be obtained from the measurement of intracardiac pressure (right ventricle or pulmonary artery). The *pulmonary capillary wedge pressure* is obtained by advancing a catheter with a balloon cuff near the tip to the pulmonary capillary bed, and then inflating the balloon so that the detecting tip detects pressures which are in close approximation to left atrial pressure. Left atrial filling pressure may be invaluable in seriously ill patients with right or left ventricular failure. It must be recognized, however, that the placement of catheters for these more advanced monitoring manoeuvres is a highly skilled practice carrying risk of serious morbidity if the technique is performed incompetently.

Even more sophisticated catheter systems allow thermal or dye detection devices which facilitate the estimation of blood flow and cardiac output.

Pulse oximetry

This measures oxygen saturation (SpO_2) of a finger tip or ear lobe, provided pulsatile blood flow is present. Pulse oximeters are robust instruments which allow continuous assessment of oxygenation for as long as the detector probe is properly placed. Pulse oximetry is invaluable in detecting patterns of desaturation, for example, in the postoperative period.

SpO_2 is not the same as arterial oxygen saturation but in many circumstances the values are very close. On the other hand it should be realized that there are many sources of error in the practice of pulse oximetry ranging from the influence of surrounding light, movement, high bilirubinaemia, a weak pulsatile flow, etc.

Gas analysers

The physical basis of *oxygen* detection and measurement may be the fuel cell or the polarograph. A discussion of these principles is beyond the scope of this book. Suffice to say that oxygen detectors are remarkably stable and robust. The presence of an oxygen monitor reassures the anaesthetist that the delivered gas composition is appropriate.

Carbon dioxide analysers allow breath-by-breath analysis of CO_2 in the respired gas. The rise and fall of CO_2 concentration as detected by a monitor is reassurance that artificial ventilation is in fact ventilating the lung alveoli (as distinct, for example, from the stomach via an inappropriately placed tracheal tube). The end tidal or highest tension or partial pressure of CO_2, reflecting the alveolar tension, is in close approximation to the PCO_2 of pulmonary capillary blood. Thus CO_2 gives a reliable indication of the adequacy or otherwise of alveolar ventilation (see Ch. 8).

Volatile anaesthetics and nitrous oxide

While the anaesthetist usually has a reasonably accurate idea of the concentration or tension of these drugs respired by the patient, the relatively inexpensive detection of these molecules allows a continuous display of the inspired and expired concentrations from the patient breathing system. The sampling point is usually at the junction of the patient airway (e.g. tracheal tube) with the delivery system from the anaesthetic machine.

In addition to the sophisticated systems that have been described above, it should be realized that much valuable information can be obtained by regular examination of the patient's skin for colour change, evidence of sweating, small muscle movement, etc. The measurement of urine output is an invaluable reassurance on the adequacy of cardiovascular function and blood volume, particularly in major surgery.

Figure 16.2 shows a typical monitor display of data on gas analysis.

Neuromuscular junction

An indicator of the effect of neuromuscular blocking drugs is the observation of muscle movement and the detection of an adequate

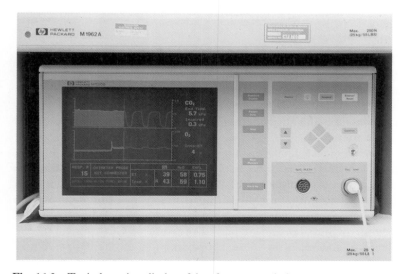

Fig. 16.2   Typical monitor display of data from gas analysis.

ventilatory pattern during recovery from neuromuscular block in anaesthesia. There is a variety of nerve stimulators providing transcutaneous stimulation of peripheral nerves with detection of response either by the naked eye or using some type of transducer. A typical arrangement involves twitch or tetanic stimulation of the ulnar nerve at the wrist with detection of a response, or non-response, in the adductor pollicis muscle, which in turn causes adduction activity of the thumb. The use of nerve stimulators is an important method for establishing that the effect of neuromuscular block has recovered sufficiently to facilitate restoration of spontaneous ventilation.

17. The anaesthetist and the management of pain

There is a need to clarify terminology. In Chapter 9, page 157, the management of *acute* pain following surgical operation is discussed; the same principles should apply for pain associated with sudden severe injury. An important development in pain relief therapy has been the recognition of ways in which techniques can be brought together for the management of what used to be called chronic pain and, in particular, the pain of cancer. Some doctors who specialize in the field of 'chronic' pain are unhappy with the term 'chronic' because it implies a pessimistic attitude which they wish to discourage. Thus it has become fashionable to refer to *pain management* or to refer specifically to cancer pain.

Chronic pain has many complex facets. Pain can induce a refractory sense of despair in the patient, coupled with an often justified feeling that the caring services have failed. These impressions are compounded if the patient knows that the end of the process is death, with possible exacerbation of the symptoms in the meantime. Over the last 20 years there has been an important development of hospices within the UK. They provide an ideal setting for bringing together the medical, nursing, psychological and spiritual needs of any patient with cancer which is likely to be terminal. The hospice concept has, of course, been extended to cater for patients with other serious conditions, notably AIDS.

Although cancer pain may account for a large proportion of the work of some pain relief specialists, there is also a need to treat other patients with longer-term pain. For example, the complex problem of back pain is endemic to western society. Indeed, the oldest surviving surgical text, the Edwin Smith papyrus of 1500 BC, describes a case of back strain. A recent UK Government report suggested that some 52 million working days were lost as the result of back pain in 1993 alone.

It is not the purpose of this book to detail any particular aspect of pain management. Rather we wish to reflect medical and social problems presented by pain in various aspects, and to list some important principles.

PAIN CLINIC

Typically this service has access, in addition to areas for consultation and examination, to operating theatre time for procedures under sedation or anaesthesia and facilities for imaging.

The case mix in pain clinics may not always be representative of the general patient population with problems. Referral depends on the particular interests and expertise of the doctors concerned. Some pain clinics are open for referral from family practitioners, some from various specialists over a wide geographical area. Yet other clinics restrict their patient intake to referrals from the particular hospital in which they are located.

In patients with cancer, pain is experienced by 20–50% at the time of diagnosis but up to 75% of patients with advanced disease. Patients with chronic non-malignant pain may be referred by general practitioners, accident and emergency departments, or by hospital specialists in almost every clinical branch of medicine.

Patients attending the pain clinic should be received in pleasant surroundings and dealt with efficiently, preferably by the same personnel on return visits. There are no reliable and validated clinical guidelines for the management of chronic pain. It is generally recommended that patients with chronic pain or cancer pain should receive individualized management usually with a combination of therapies given simultaneously. The basic modalities are:

Prevention. Early active rehabilitation should be encouraged wherever possible and this will reduce the occurrence of chronic disability following an episode of low back pain. The likelihood of chronic pain after nerve injury or nerve damage may be lessened by an effective early management regimen.

Medication. Conventional analgesics and a wide range of other drugs are prescribed for chronic pain but convincing evidence from controlled trials is lacking in most instances.

Peripheral nerve blocks, epidural and facet joint injections and sympathetic ganglion blockade for intravenous regional blocks are all used for chronic pain and cancer pain treatment. The substances injected include local anaesthetics, neurolytic solutions such as phenol or alcohol, and steroids. There is a variety of physical methods for ablating nerves including cryolesions or radiofrequency thermocoagulation.

Transcutaneous electrical nerve stimulation (TENS) is a form of peripheral nerve or spinal cord stimulation which, by activating 'gate' mechanisms within the central nervous system, may lead to the 'shutting off' of pain stimuli from the periphery.

Neurosurgery. Very occasionally surgical procedures to divide neural pathways may prove effective in pain relief. It is important to stress, however, that surgical intervention is efficacious in only a small minority of carefully chosen patients.

Other supportive manoeuvres. Physiotherapy, including exercises and manipulation, may offer effective rehabilitation in some patients. Psychological and behavioural approaches may be useful in many patients with chronic non-malignant pain and some forms of pain resulting from cancer.

A task force of the International Association for the Study of Pain (IASP) has defined the desirable resource for pain treatment facilities. A multidisciplinary approach is recommended wherever possible so that a suitable range of disciplines can be available for both diagnosis and treatment of pain problems. It is recognized, of course, that not every patient requires an interdisciplinary approach.

Appendix

SI units

The International System of Units (Système International, SI) was adopted in 1960 by the General Conference of Weights and Measures as a logical, coherent system based on seven fundamental units: metre, kilogram, second, ampere, kelvin, candela and mole.

The system has been adopted generally by international scientific bodies, including the International Federation of Clinical Chemistry (IFCC) and the Section of Clinical Chemistry of the International Union of Pure and Applied Chemistry (IUPAC).

All measurements are expressed in the basic units or in units derived from them. The seven basic units, and some of the derived units relevant to medicine, with standard abbreviations are:

Physical quantity	Name of SI unit	Symbol
Length	metre	m
Mass	kilogram	kg
Time	second	s
Electric current	ampere	A
Temperature	kelvin	K
Luminous intensity	candela	cd
Amount of substance	mole	mol
Energy	joule	J
Force	newton	N
Power	watt	W
Pressure	pascal	Pa

Prefixes to indicate fractions or multiples of the basic or derived units have also been defined.

Prefixes for SI units

Factor	Name	Symbol	Factor	Name	Symbol
10^{18}	exa-	E	10^{-18}	atto-	a
10^{15}	peta-	P	10^{-15}	femto-	f
10^{12}	tera-	T	10^{-12}	pico-	p
10^{9}	giga-	G	10^{-9}	nano-	n
10^{6}	mega-	M	10^{-6}	micro-	μ
10^{3}	kilo-	k	10^{-3}	milli-	m
10^{2}	hecto-	h	10^{-2}	centi-	c
10	deca-	da	10^{-1}	deci-	d

Index